THE PRACTICAL BOOK OF
COLOR THERAPY

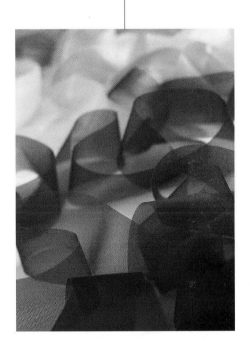

THE PRACTICAL BOOK OF
COLOR THERAPY

STEP-BY-STEP TECHNIQUES TO HARNESS THE HEALING POWERS OF LIGHT AND COLOR SHOWN IN OVER 250 PHOTOGRAPHS

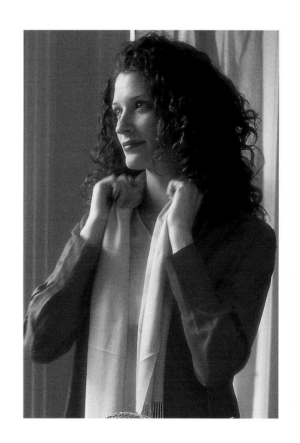

SUSAN LILLY AND SIMON LILLY

southwater

This edition is published by Southwater, an imprint of Anness Publishing Ltd, Hermes House, 88–89 Blackfriars Road, London SE1 8HA; tel. 020 7401 2077; fax 020 7633 9499

www.southwaterbooks.com; www.annesspublishing.com

If you like the images in this book and would like to investigate using them for publishing, promotions or advertising, please visit our website www.practicalpictures.com for more information.

UK agent: The Manning Partnership Ltd; tel. 01225 478444; fax 01225 478440; sales@manning-partnership.co.uk

UK distributor: Book Trade Services; tel. 0116 2759086; fax 0116 2759090; uksales@booktradeservices.com; exportsales@booktradeservices.com

North American agent/distributor: National Book Network; tel. 301 459 3366; fax 301 429 5746; www.nbnbooks.com

Australian agent/distributor: Pan Macmillan Australia; tel. 1300 135 113; fax 1300 135 103; customer.service@macmillan.com.au

New Zealand agent/distributor: David Bateman Ltd; tel. (09) 415 7664; fax (09) 415 8892

Publisher: Joanna Lorenz
Managing Editor: Helen Sudell
Senior Editor: Joanne Rippin
Special photography: Michelle Garrett
Designer: Nigel Partridge
Editorial Reader: Diane Ashmore
Production Controller: Claire Rae

ETHICAL TRADING POLICY
Because of our ongoing ecological investment program, you, as our customer, can have the pleasure and reassurance of knowing that a tree is being cultivated on your behalf to naturally replace the materials used to make the book you are holding. For further information about this scheme, go to www.annesspublishing.com/trees

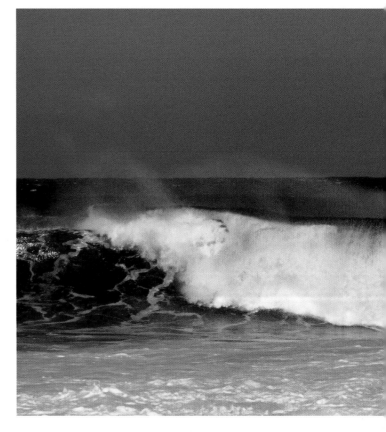

A CIP catalogue record for this book is available from the British Library.

Previously published as *The Power of Color and Color Healing*

PUBLISHER'S NOTE
Although the advice and information in this book are believed to be accurate and true at the time of going to press, neither the authors nor the publisher can accept any legal responsibility or liability for any errors or omissions that may be made.
This book is not intended to replace advice from a qualified medical practitioner. Please seek a medical opinion if you have any concerns about your health. Neither the authors nor the publishers can accept any liability for failure to follow this advice.

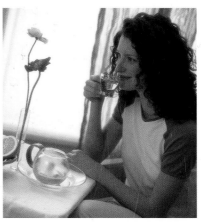

Contents

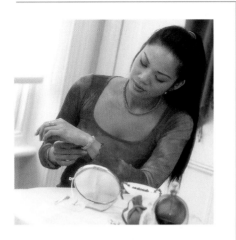

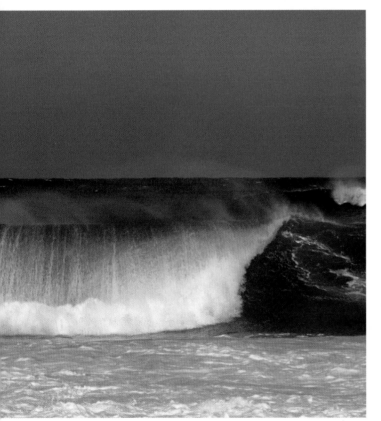

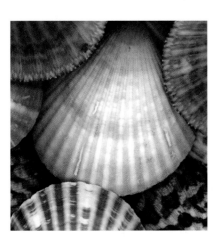

introduction

Our sense of sight is our primary interaction with the world around us, but we take that process almost for granted. We rarely stop to think about what is happening when we see colour, what colour means to us and how it might affect us in many different ways.

Light is a form of energy and all energy acts on the matter that it comes into contact with. What we see as colour is simply the brain's way of recognizing the many different energy qualities of light.

When sunlight passes into our atmosphere from space, its rate of vibration, or frequency, is altered slightly. Our eyes identify this frequency change as a shift of colour: if the frequency slows down we perceive a shift towards the red end of the spectrum, if the frequency is speeded up we see it as a shift towards the cooler, blue end of the spectrum. This effect is seen by the eye and brain when light passes through any substance that changes its frequency of vibration. We tend to think of colour as existing on surfaces, but the colour of an object is determined by what happens to the light that hits it. The colour we see, very often, is exactly what that object is not.

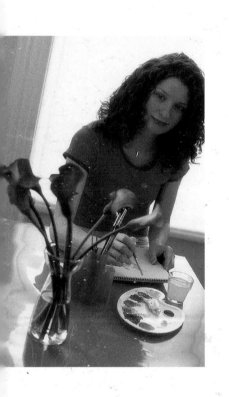

Every frequency of visible light, each colour, creates changes in us at all levels, physically, emotionally and mentally. Different cultures have given different attributes and meanings to colour, but at the biological level we all react in the same way. Colour is not superficial or ephemeral. Colour shows us the energetic reality of the world around us. Learning to recognize and use colour with awareness can bring positive and powerful changes into our lives.

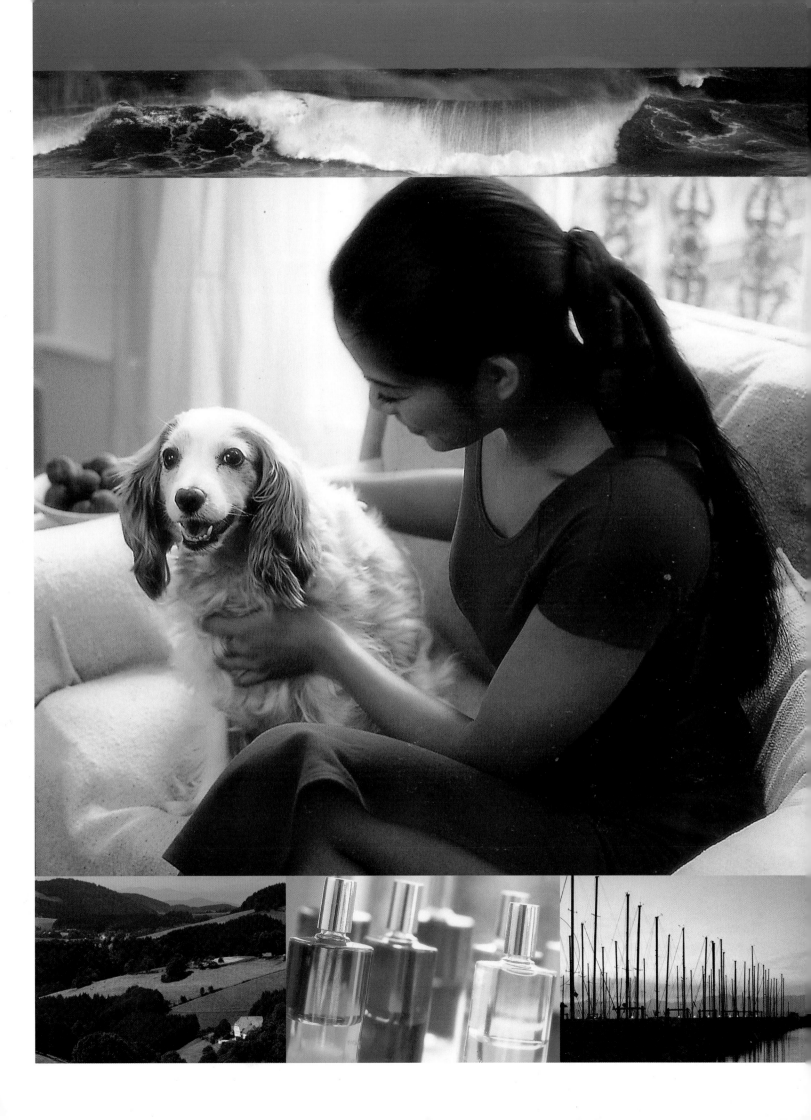

The Fundamentals of Colour

Colour is a universal language. Everything under the sun is affected by colour. Plants, animals, bacteria, chemical reactions, all exhibit changes of behaviour when exposed to different colours. It is also a subconscious language that we use instinctively in every area of our lives.

Natural environments

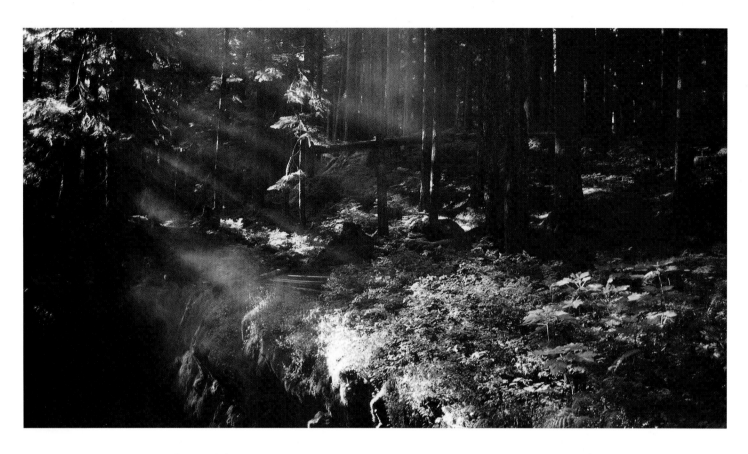

The human characteristic of adaptability allows us to successfully inhabit all sorts of environments. Whether living in a forest or a desert, people adapt to the unique qualities of their surroundings. We get used to the colours and shapes around us, which is why a change of scene, such as a holiday, makes us sharply, refreshingly aware of many different details of colour, light and shape. Colour plays a big part in creating the ambience and mood of a place because its vibrational energy charges our emotions and energy levels.

the calm of nature

When escaping from the crowded and grey environment of towns and cities, most people experience a noticeable relaxation and lifting of mood as the green of nature fills their vision. Walking through woodland where the light is predominantly filtered through green leaves creates a sense of calm in the emotions and an expansive, increased sense of connection with our surroundings.

△ **Inside a wood or forest the trees alter the quality of light to something completely different from the one that exists outside it.**

The feeling of relaxation and the renewed sense of mental perspective during and after a country walk is so common that few will stop to think about it when the walk is over, but they will subconsciously feel profound benefits from the experience.

holiday happiness

Many people enjoy relaxing by the seaside in summer. The predominant colours are the blues of the sea and sky, which introduce a feeling of expansiveness and peace. Turquoise tempers the deeper blues with an extra sense of calm and comfort. The golden yellow of sand and sunlight energize the body's systems, helping to restore balanced functioning by reducing anxiety and stress levels, and creating happiness and clarity in the mind. It is no wonder with today's hectic lifestyle that two weeks doing

▽ **When we dream of holidays, the first image that often comes to mind is a beach. The yellows and blues of the seaside revitalize our energies.**

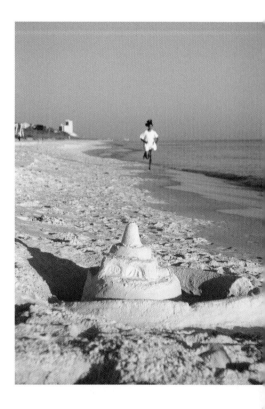

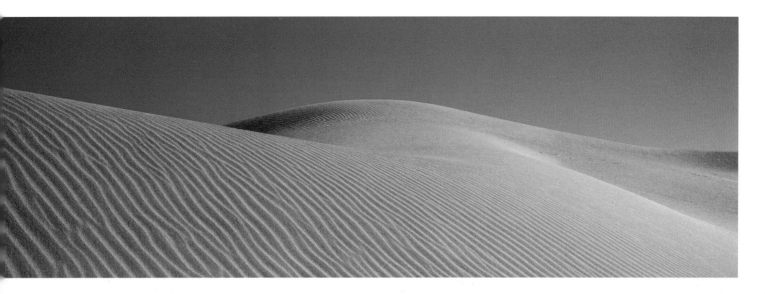

the fundamentals of colour

△ Deserts provide endless variations of a few colours and their calm stillness has inspired visionaries and mystics for centuries.

special places

Colour in the landscape separates and defines special places. The white cliffs of Dover symbolize more than simply the end of the land of England. Their very starkness suggests both a barrier of otherworldliness, a mystical separation from the mainland of Europe – and, when seen from afar – an invitation to explore new possibilities.

In Australia, Uluru (Ayer's Rock) is sacred to the Aborigine peoples, not just because of its shape and size, but because of the amazing red coloration the rock has, especially at sunset. The colour of blood, the energy of life and heat, it rises dramatically out of the vast landscape and is regarded by the Aboriginals as the birthplace of the gods. In the south-west states of America, the canyons, especially the Painted Canyon, were held in the same awe by the people living in the region because the powerful colour symbolism was so suggestive of the generative forces of life. In the same way certain mountains – Mt Shasta in California, Mt Fuji in Japan and Mt Kailash in the Tibetan Himalayas – are held in awe as focuses of power and transcendence because their white peaks dominate the landscape and evoke the purity of the heavenly realms.

▽ Uluru, formerly known as Ayer's Rock, in Australia is a perfect example of how the natural colour of rock can take on magical and sacred significance for the people who live near it.

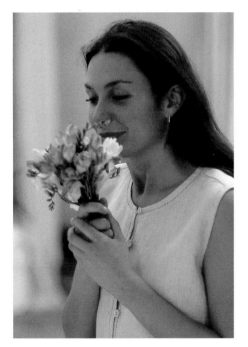

△ Archaeological evidence shows that our earliest ancestors felt exactly the same as we do about flowers, offering tokens made from them at important ceremonies and life-events.

nothing and simply being on a beach in the sunshine is regarded by many as the perfect holiday, and one which they will repeat each year with unfailing regularity.

The same colour combination of blues and golds occurs in many desert or near-desert conditions and it is perhaps significant that in the past many people have sought the deserts of the world as places of mysticism, for contemplation, visions and religious inspiration. With such isolation, very few distractions and the stimulus of blues, golds and yellows directly affecting the function of the nervous system, such places encourage the deepest thought.

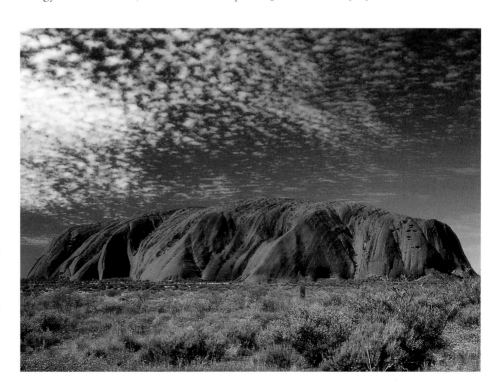

Nature's use of colour

In the natural world colour is used in two main ways: to hide and to reveal. Considering that full colour vision is a very rare development in the animal world it is surprising how sophisticated nature's use of colour can be.

the seeing world

In the simplest of eyes there is only the ability to distinguish between light and dark. In creatures that live in darkness, for example in the depths of the ocean, colour vision is not as important as other sensory mechanisms for identifying electromagnetic radiations such as electric currents. But where there is sunlight, colour vision does become important. Experiments have shown that though many insects are sensitive only to green, blue and violet light, they can see beyond the human range, well into ultraviolet. Birds, dogs and cats have different degrees of colour recognition depending on the importance of sight

▽ The courtship and mating rituals of birds rely heavily on dramatic displays of colour in the male's plumage.

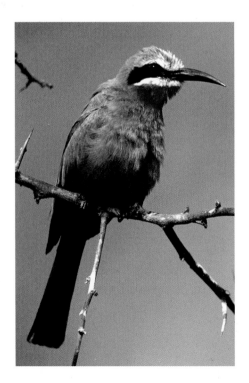

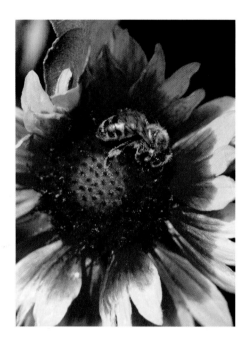

△ Bees' eyes see different frequencies of light from those that the human eye is able to recognize. Ultraviolet frequencies play a vital role in the bee's ability to locate flowers.

compared with their other sensing mechanisms. Owls and hawks need acute visual sensitivity to movement, while dogs rely less on colour vision because their highly effective sense of smell is their dominant sense for gathering information. Full-spectrum colour is seen by the higher vertebrates, including humans, as well as a few unexpected animals, such as tortoises and the octopus.

The eye is not the only mechanism for recording light and colour, nor does the greatest use of colour belong to those creatures with the best colour vision. The eye is simply a specialist organ for recording colour and light. Light is an energy and its vibrations can create many changes in physical matter. It is thought that within the human skin there are specialist cells that have a great sensitivity to light, and that it is possible to notice subtle changes that take place when these are exposed to colours. It seems that this method of sensing increases when there is impairment of vision.

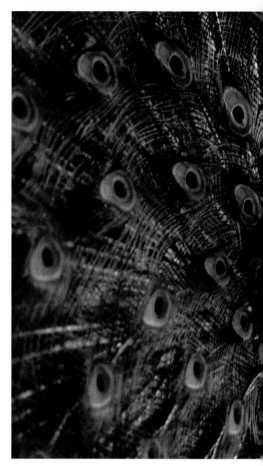

△ The male peacock has evolved a fabulous display of tail feathers to attract a mate.

Plants have no specialized organs for colour recognition as such, yet colour is employed magnificently as a communication device. Bees and other insects are drawn to flowers by their colour and this ensures the fertilization of seeds and the continuation of the species. As it ripens, fruit accumulates sugars, so changing colour to indicate that it has become edible to animals. The animals then eat the fruit and spread the seeds through their droppings.

▽ Some animals use colour to imitate aggressive species as a form of protection. Some butterflies, for example, have large eye-like markings.

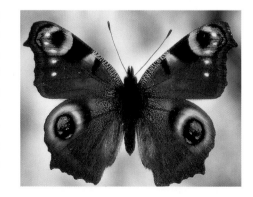

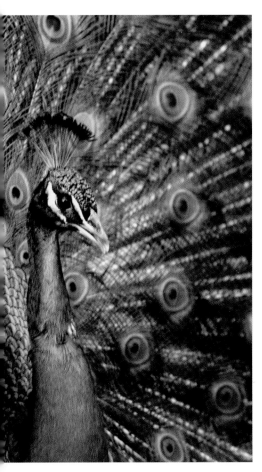

colour prevailing in a habitat. So, for example, the ragged vertical stripes of the zebra help it to blend into the tall grasses of the African plains, by disguising its size and shape. Some creatures have the ability to change colour very quickly, to achieve an almost perfect match with their background. The slow-moving chameleon has an amazing range of colour changes as does the bottom-feeding flatfish, the plaice. Both of these creatures are virtually impossible to see until they move. Perhaps the most unusual and striking use of colour is the protective warning or camouflage device of the squid, which has evolved a complex and beautiful language of expression and mood by sending constantly changing waves of rippling colours across its body.

▽ No colouring is accidental or superficial, it is a survival strategy, an evolutionary advantage that all creatures, such as this jellyfish, utilize.

warning signals

In some creatures bright and striking colour displays are used to attract a mate or to act as a warning of aggressive superiority. The male peacock displays its fan of wonderful tail feathers when trying to attract the attentions of a female and to demonstrate superiority to a potential rival. In insects and snakes, bold, distinctive markings, such as the yellow and black stripes of the wasp, are recognized as danger signals by other species. This colour strategy can be so effective that even some completely non-toxic and harmless animals mimic the coloration of a poisonous or dangerous species to avoid unwanted attention from predators. The eye and face patterns on the wings of some butterflies and moths mimic the aggressive displays of much larger animals to much the same effect.

camouflage

Using colour to blend with the surroundings is a common strategy. Camouflage often mimics the light and

▷ The chameleon has developed special pigment cells that rapidly blend with its surroundings to disguise it from predators who rely on sight.

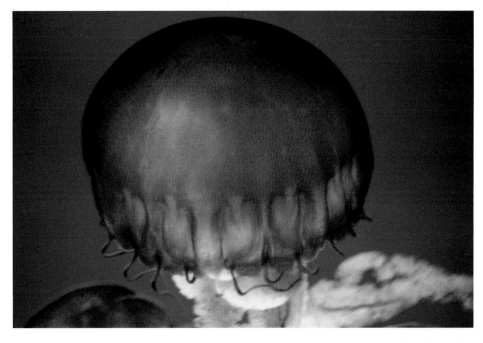

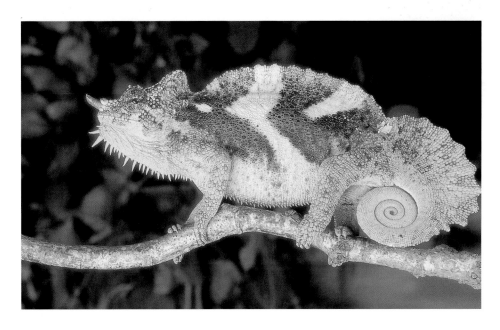

Cultural variations

Although the physical effects of colour are biologically constant, people living in different climates understand and interpret colour in ways that can differ, and even oppose each other. Colour becomes a language of tribe and culture, which may mean little or nothing to outsiders. The energy of colour remains the same but the significance of that energy changes.

black and white

For people of the northern hemisphere, the north is a region of ice and snow where the sun never travels. The north therefore is associated with the white of snow or the black of winter and night. In the southern hemisphere, however, winter weather comes

▽ Depending on geographical position white is associated with either the north or the south.

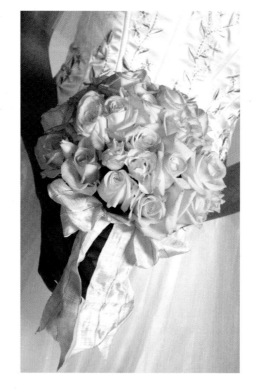

◁ White has become traditional for Western weddings where it is regarded as a symbol of purity and new beginnings.

from Antarctica, from the south, and therefore white and black are linked to the south rather than the north. This affects other colours and elements accordingly.

In Europe, for example, death has traditionally been associated with the colour black. Funeral cortèges use black cars, and coffin bearers and mourners dress in black. In China, however, mourners wear white, because white is the colour of winter when all things return to the earth in a dormant state. In fact, traditionally minded Chinese will avoid wearing white, because it reminds them of the death shroud, whereas in the West, white is associated with innocence.

red and white

There are some colour combinations that seem to have the same resonance across most of the world. Two of the colours most

▽ Father Christmas reflects the role of shaman in many of his characteristics.

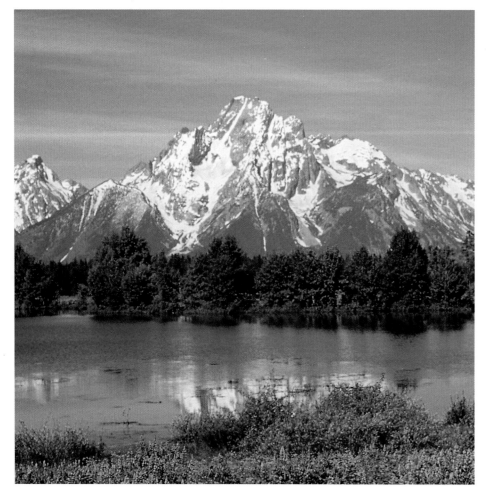

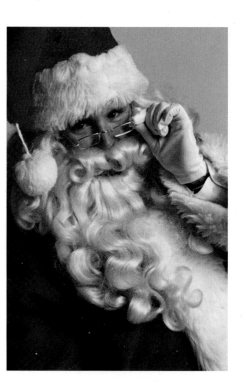

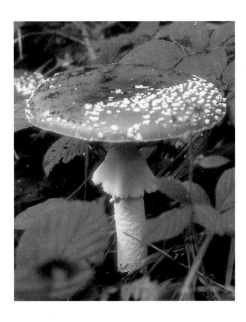

◁ The colours of the fly agaric mushroom drew attention to its magical properties, and it still symbolizes fairyland in children's stories.

▽ In this Navajo sand painting, every colour used is as symbolic as the complex imagery that is held in its design.

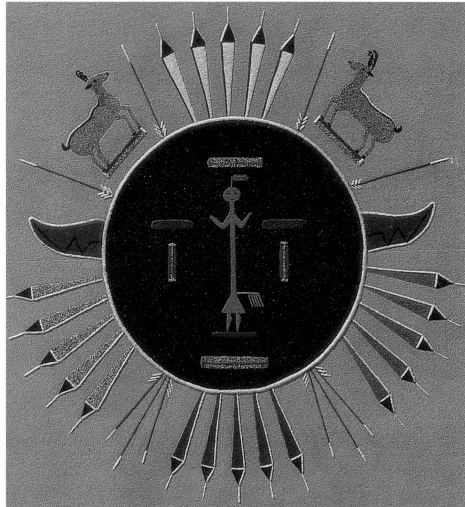

frequently found together are red and white, symbolizing the polarities of male and female. In Tibetan symbolism and in some pagan traditions, red is the colour of the female Sun, white the male Moon. The two together are the power of creation, the union of opposites, the joining of Heaven and Earth. Right across the northern hemisphere, in the Arctic and temperate zones, these colours appear each autumn after the fertilizing rains, in the form of the fly agaric mushroom, with its red top and white spots. The fly agaric is a favourite food of the reindeer of Lapland, and the native

▽ Each figure in this Tibetan mandala is identified by its colour, denoting the exact energy each manifestation displays to the meditator.

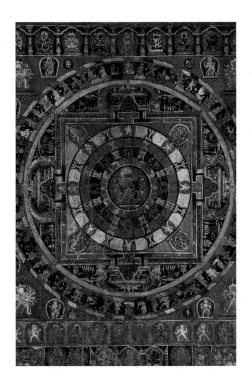

Sami peoples of that region observed the apparent intoxication that the animals showed after eating the fungi. The Sami, along with every Siberian tribe, woodland American Indians and others, learned to dry and eat small portions of the mushroom in order to enter exalted altered states of reality, the realms of the spirits and gods. Ceremonial costumes of red, decorated with white polka dots, are worn by the shamans and healers of these peoples even today.

It is interesting that the Western image of Father Christmas retains all the symbolism of the Arctic shaman: dressed in red and white, he is drawn in his sleigh by reindeer, and he travels across the sky-worlds to bring the magic of gifts to his people in their time of hardship – the depths of winter.

green

In Western Europe forests dominated the landscape for thousands of years. The colour green was always associated with the wildness of nature, the power of growth and of freedom. The woodland world was believed to be inhabited by spirits, elves and fairies, who were often dressed in green. The dominant energy, the intelligence of nature, was represented by the Green Man – a fusion of human and plant life. In the Arabic world, the colour green is the sacred colour of Islam. In a landscape dominated by desert and arid wilderness, green represents oases, which give life, food, water and shelter. To the Arabic mind, green is the refuge of heavenly paradise. For the West, green is the force of worldly nature.

the fundamentals of colour

Mankind's use of colour has developed from the needs and limitations of the environment. The first colours used were the earth colours – the red, ochre and black of cave paintings created from ground-up iron-bearing rocks and clays, and soot. Red ochre is known to have been the earliest dye used on a worldwide scale, and sacred red is found in burial chambers in most parts of the world.

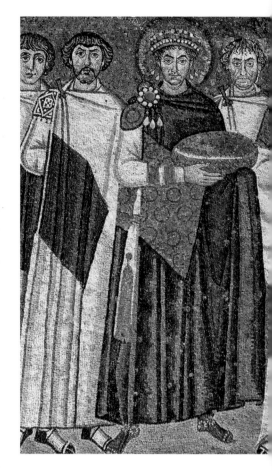

◁ Metallic oxides have been an important source of natural colours, often proving more stable than vegetable dyes and with richer colours.

development of dyes

Plant dyes provide a good range of browns, yellows, blues and greens. The rarity of a colour or the difficulty of producing a dye quickened the birth of the fashion industry. Only rich or powerful individuals were able to use expensive colours, which then became symbols of privilege and power. Blue was difficult to produce so the plant woad was precious and its use probably had spiritual significance to the ancient Britons and Picts who were famed for its use. In the long history of the Roman Empire, the most prestigious colour was purple, extracted from the shells of Mediterranean shellfish, by a secret process originally known only to the Phoenician traders of the eastern seaboard. Wearing purple robes was the exclusive right of the emperor. Lesser nobles were ranked by the precise widths of purple stripe that they were allowed to wear on their togas. Wearing too much purple was a serious offence.

display and concealment

Colour is used in dress both to display and to conceal, just as it is in nature. Tartans show a complex intermingling of the practical and social uses of colour. Examples of woven tartans have been found on mummies in the Taklamakan desert of Mongolia, though today this cloth is more often associated with Scotland and Ireland.

The exact choice and blend of colours as well as the pattern of warp and weave in Scottish tartans are unique to each clan or tribal grouping, and no one would dream of wearing another clan's tartan. Every tartan also has several variations of colour and pattern – for example, the hunting and dress tartans. Hunting tartans use a subtle blend of tones to act as an effective camouflage in the Highland landscape. Dress tartans have more showy colours, with bright red and yellows in contrasting bands, and are worn at social and formal occasions.

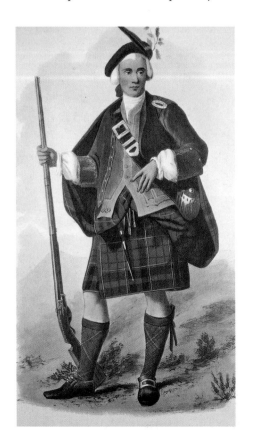

◁ Tartan shows a classic use of the way colour can identify a group of people by what they wear.

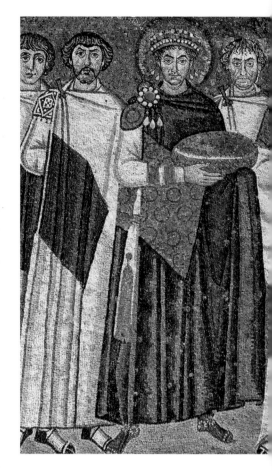

△ In this Byzantine mosaic each figure's rank and status is identified by the amount of purple worn. The central figure is the Emperor Justinian, dressed all in purple.

▽ Bold colours and extravagant designs have characterized war dress for millennia. Colour is used to threaten the opposition and create a sense of unity among warriors on the same side.

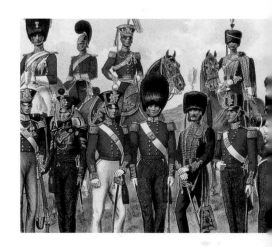

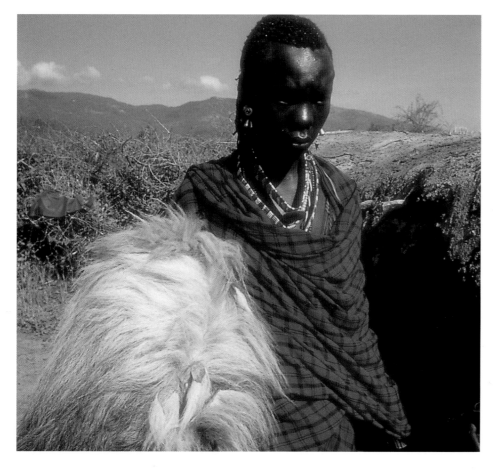

modern fashion industry also offers a sense of group identity and status, while giving the illusion of personal expression in style or colour. Though synthetic dyes have widened the palette of colours enormously, the fashion industry, working three seasons ahead, dictates which shades of what colour are going to be in the shops for us to buy.

colour in clothes today

By becoming more aware of the message colour gives out, it is possible to change from hunter to warrior, from belonging to standing alone, from being lost in the crowd to being an individual. For people living in the West, this becomes more difficult when limited to the styles and colours available in stores. In parts of the world where hand-woven fabric and handmade clothes are still common, the messages of colour are clearer, and are easily read on a subconscious level.

▽ There is now a vast range of colours available in fabrics, thanks to synthetic dyes.

△ The Maasai tribe in East Africa favour a bright red dye for their robes.

◁ In Peru traditional clothing tends to be as bright and colourful as possible.

group identity

While the hunter always favours subtle camouflaging colours, the warrior aims at maximum display. Colour becomes not only an identification, but also an aggressive statement, and therefore red is a common military colour. The bright red uniform that the British Infantry wore for hundreds of years was worn to intimidate. Other groups, such as the Maasai, also dress warriors in red.

Traditional clothing around the world tends to reflect the unity of the tribal group. The outsider may perceive all members of the group as dressing alike, but there will usually be subtle differences that clearly denote rank and status to the insider. The

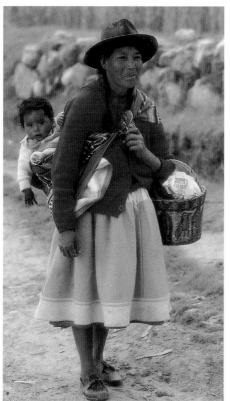

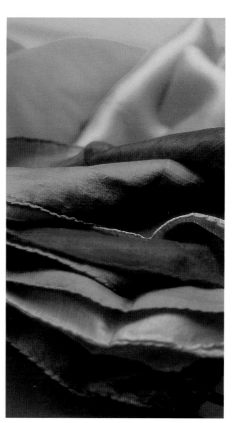

Colour co-ordination

An instinct for harmonizing and co-ordinating colour is a gift that some people are born with, but the rest of us can manage if we follow a few guidelines. In practice, shades, tones and tints that work well together do so because of their natural visual relationship, and there are simple rules to mixing and matching colour.

When similar colours are placed next to each other, each loses some of its vibrant qualities. Complementary colours, those opposite to each other on the colour wheel, will augment each other's qualities. Colours that are next but one to each other on the

▽ Colour in nature, designed for survival, often makes harmonious juxtapositions that are borrowed by fashion designers.

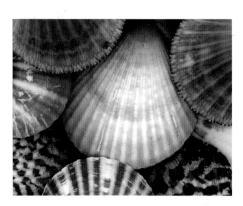

▷ The colour wheel here is often described as the True Colour Wheel. This presentation of colour was put together by Sir Isaac Newton and has been used by many famous colour workers, such as Goethe and Steiner. It shows the complementary colour to red as turquoise. In the Artist's Colour Wheel, not shown here, the complementary colour to red is shown as green.

HOW COLOURS ARE DEFINED

- A hue is the quality of a colour that enables us to classify it as red, green, yellow etc.
- A tint is a hue with white added.
- A shade is a hue with black added.
- A tone is a hue with grey added. Tints look good together, as do shades or tones, but mixing tints, shades and tones does not always work well.

True Colour Wheel, present pleasing combinations that are often employed as tints by interior designers to create a comfortable space.

colour categories

Carol Jackson, the author of the book *Colour Me Beautiful*, formulated categories of colour into a practical and easy to use system, based upon the four elements (fire, earth, air and water) and the seasons (spring, summer, autumn and winter). She applied the colour groupings to décor, furnishings, clothes and make-up.

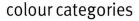

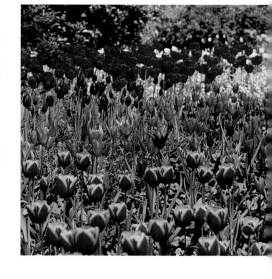

△ Plants naturally grow together in swathes of the same species. Garden designers develop this theme of group planting to create stunning displays.

Spring colours are those linked to the water element. They feature warm and light tints, and no dark colours. Spring colours include turquoise, lilac, peach, coral, scarlet, violet, emerald, sunshine yellow, cream and sand. All the colours in this category are clear and almost delicate. They create a joyful and nurturing ambience.

Summer colours, linked to the air element, are all tones (that is, they have a lot of grey in them). This range of colours is

▽ Colours that are familiar to each season's changes become associated with the qualities of that time of year, and are reflected in our clothes.

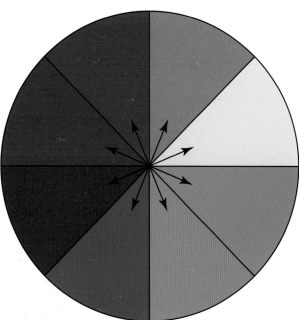

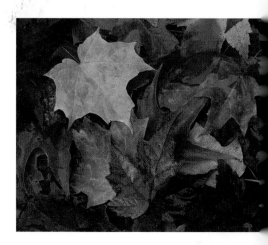

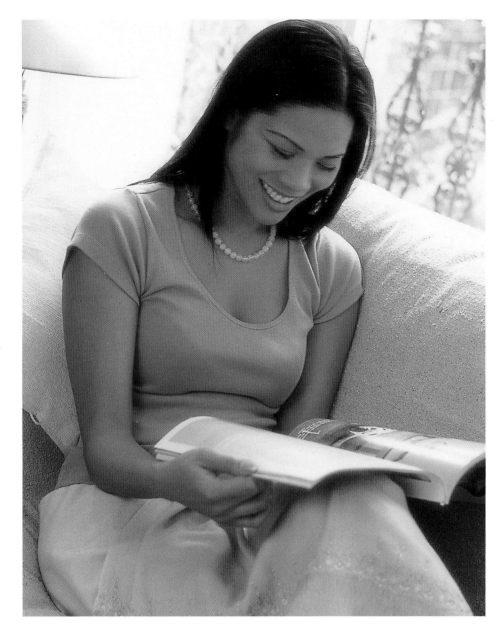

◁ When it comes to choices in fashion, no one system will suit everyone. Colouring and personality are factors to consider but the colours should also 'feel' right to wear.

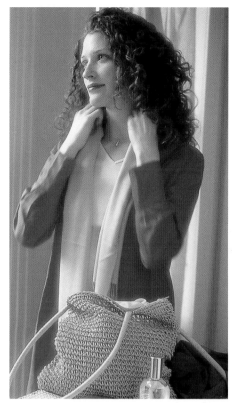

△ Experiment with a wide range of colours in your clothing, and don't be afraid to mix strong shades together if that's what feels right.

▽ Try dressing in a colour range that complements your natural colouring and also dress in a contrasting style to compare. See how your behaviour is modified.

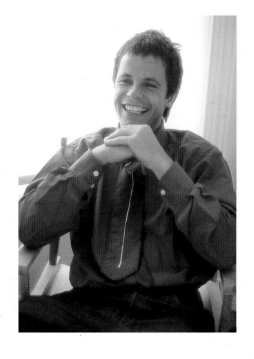

very subtle and includes maroon, rose, powder blue, sage green, pale yellow, lavender, plum, oyster and taupe. This is a 'middle-of-the-road' selection, that includes darker colours, but not heavy colours. Summer colours have an elegance that is also cool and contained.

Autumn colours are related to the fire element. These are warm colours. All are shades, which means they have black in them. They include mustard, olive green, flame, peacock, burnt orange, teal and burgundy. These colours are very rich and striking. They suggest maturity and depth.

Winter colours are connected with the earth element and feature a big contrast between hues, tints and shades. Winter colours include black, white, magenta, cyan, purple, lemon, silver, indigo, royal blue and jade. None of these colours are subtle, they are all bold and powerful.

These colour groupings can also reflect psychological personality types, not simply a person's natural colouring or skin type. For example, winter colours are often favoured by people with strong business sense, confidence and a practical nature. Spring colours, on the other hand, are popular with those of an artistic, sensitive and quiet disposition.

There can also be a strong second preference in colour groupings. Occasionally the second preference can be useful in choosing clothes that are designed to create a particular effect, for a presentation or interview for example. However, wearing colours to impress people may feel rather uncomfortable compared to wearing your natural, instinctive choice. Both men and women can use these colour categories for choosing clothes, and women often use it too when selecting make-up.

Colour for commercial use

Colour affects everyone at an unconscious level, that is, below the awareness of normal everyday thought. So politicians, businesses and advertisers have learned to manipulate the desired response by using the language of colour. Careful use of colour can bypass the viewer's ability to discriminate or make instant critical judgements.

advertising

The human eye can distinguish between hundreds of shades of colour, and each shade elicits a slightly different emotional and behavioural response. The advertising industry exploits this ability and constantly bombards us with subliminal messages through the use of colour. As those who work with hypnosis and auto-suggestion know well, subliminal messages, because they are not recognized by the conscious mind, can have a profound effect on our behaviour and attitudes. It is the advertisers' job to select the most appropriate colours for their product 'message' as well as an image that is uniquely identifiable. The right colour or combination of colours can make all the difference to product sales.

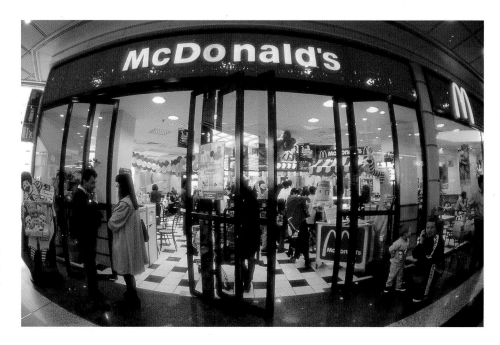

△ **Retail outlets depend on being seen and recognized. Colours and logos that can be seen from a long way have a distinct advantage.**

▽ **An effective interior design will match the colour and shape of a room to its function, creating an ideal atmosphere. Muted colours and soft lighting will promote relaxation in this restaurant's customers.**

colour manipulation

Red is the key colour in products that suggest energy, vigour, excitement and speed. Fast food outlets very often combine a bright red with yellow or white in their logos and décor. Bright yellow stimulates the digestive system, so we feel hungry, while white combined with red suggests clean, efficient service. Using bright red and a creamy white as interior colours in eating places ensures that customers are focused on the business of eating rather than on socializing. Whites and greys also prevent people from relaxing and becoming too comfortable. On the other hand, in up-market restaurants, dark, rich reds are often combined with subdued lighting to create an atmosphere of comfort and security. This encourages people to talk quietly or intimately, while taking time over a meal. Orange or yellow walls in eating places make for a convivial and a lively atmosphere, with more bustle and noise. These colours are often used in bars, bistros and coffee houses to create an ideal atmosphere for chatter and socializing.

Blue suggests sobriety, control and responsibility, and is used in products where a sense of stability and authority is required.

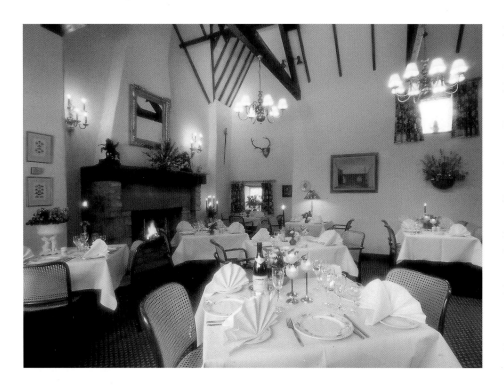

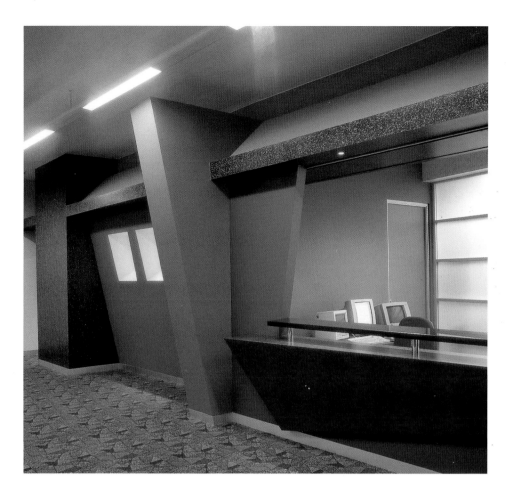

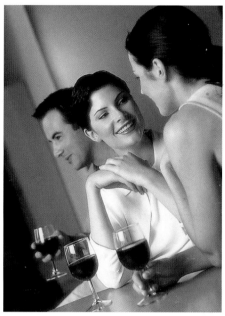

◁ This interior, though at first glance, abstract and random, draws the eye to a reception area by using warm, more welcoming colours.

▽ Warm colours in a bar setting often encourage relaxation and enjoyment.

Light or mid-blue is rarely used in food advertising as we tend to associate it with decay in that context. Dark blue labelling combined with a rich yellow or gold is often effective in the promotion of specialist gourmet foods, suggesting a certain level of detachment and even superiority from the everyday. The qualities associated with blue make it a popular colour for the interiors of public service buildings such as banks, where it helps to keep a subdued, serious and unemotional ambience.

Green colours and tones are used to promote products that suggest freshness, and naturalness. Often green coloured packaging will form part of a claim made by the manufactuer that the product will bring health benefits. Dark greens and mid tones are used in preference to olive and yellow greens, as these lighter green colours may suggest and even at times create feelings of unease and nausea.

colour at work

There is ample evidence, both anecdotal and researched, that colour is an important factor in every environment. The same pale greens that can suggest nausea in food environments, especially the sallower shades,

are often used in large public meeting spaces and corridors where people need to be encouraged to keep on the move rather than loiter and socialize. The wrong colour combinations in an office, greys and cool blues for example, or browns and tans, not

▽ In this office colours have been kept cool to encourage quiet efficiency, but avoid the sedating effect of dark blues.

only affect the mood of the staff but can also reduce profits, while creams and pale tones can create a rather uninvolved attitude from the workforce. Yellows, oranges and peachy pinks with turquoise and warm shades of green can transform a company's workforce and productivity from mediocre to efficient.

Colour should never be thoughtlessly applied. It is a vibrant, life-sustaining energy that should be used with care and skill.

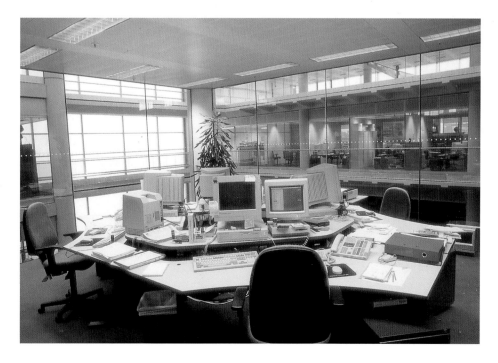

Colour inside the home

The home, whatever its shape and size, always becomes a reflection of the people who live in it. Our own space speaks volumes about our personal tastes and attitudes. Becoming more conscious of the effects of colour on behaviour, and learning what colours reflect our own energies, makes us better able to choose the right colours for our home.

Recommendations about using colour in the home, like all opinions of what is considered fashionable, are usually very culturally specific and change from one year to the next. Formulas can be helpful, but

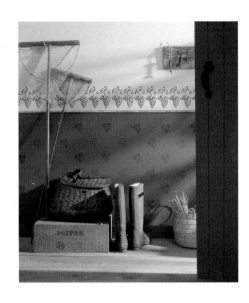

△ Tints of orange, creams and browns create a spacious feel while bringing a quality of warmth.

they should never supersede personal choice. In general, colours with red in them will warm up a cool space, such as a north-facing room. Warm colours will also make a space feel smaller. Colours with blues in them will make a room feel cool and appear larger. Dark hues will reduce the apparent size of the space and light hues will make it seem larger than it is.

entrance halls

Hallways are the first rooms entered in many homes. They are rarely large enough to be a living space and so can be treated as a transition between the outside world and the inner privacy of the rooms beyond. Hallways immediately reflect how we wish to be seen by the world. They can be extremely formal or simply act as a storage space. Colours here will suggest whether the hall is a barrier or a welcome sign. White or cream is often chosen as a neutral colour that acts as an emotional air-lock. Rich, deep colours, whether warm or cool, will create a strong impression of personality and a clear boundary to demarcate territory.

The colour used in an entrance hall will directly affect the visitor, so choose wisely. Strong reds are energizing while slightly

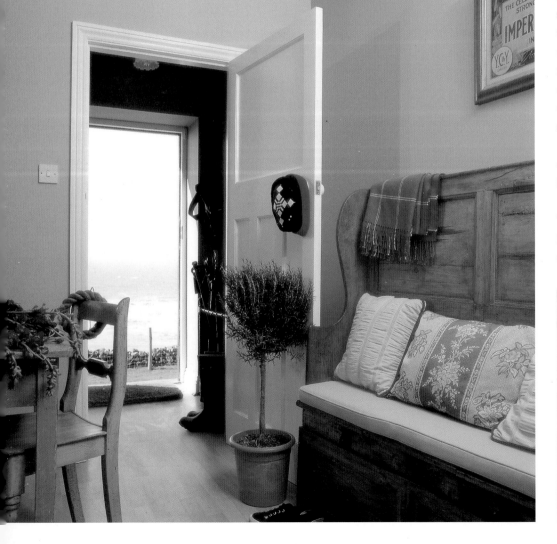

▽ Subdued earth tones are enlivened here with the use of complementary blues and yellows.

▽ The cool blues here create spaciousness and neatness. Stairs and banisters in red and yellow articulate depth and distance in a practical way.

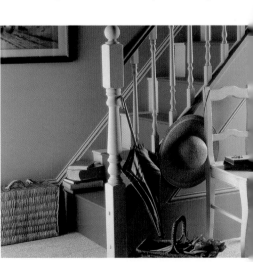

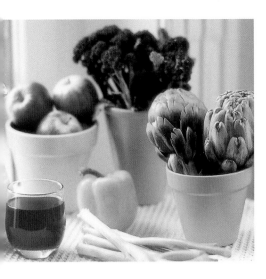

△ A mix of yellow and green items in a kitchen that is decorated in neutral colours creates a bright and cheerful room.

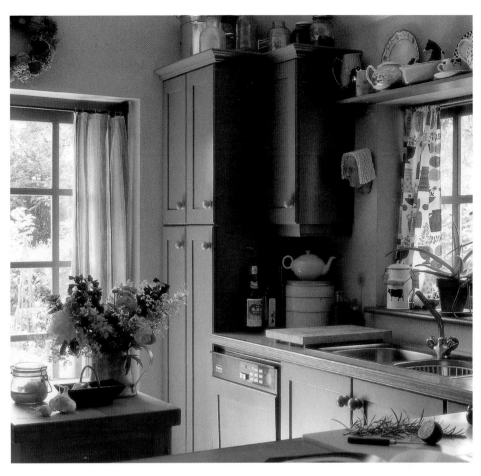

muted reds (with a hint of brown) suggest solid, powerful and practical comfort. Pinks, depending on the tint, offer a warm, friendly, non-threatening atmosphere. Blues are calming and sedating, useful for city homes where the outside world is noisy and hectic. A deep blue will help to cool over-stressed and over-stimulated nervous systems, generating relaxation and a sense of peace and quiet. Greens and browns suggest the natural world, though here it is very important which shades and tones are used. A strong, bright green can look fine in nature where light levels are so complex that they create a huge variety of subtle shades. Follow nature's example and imitate the diffusion of light by using a range of tones and shades of greens, rather than one strong block of colour.

kitchens and bathrooms

Utilitarian rooms like the kitchen and bathroom need colours that harmonize with their functions. For example, it is a good idea for bathrooms to be painted in warm tones – yellows, pinks and oranges. These give a comfortable, relaxing brightness and reflect the energies of cleansing and caring. Yellow in the kitchen, on the other hand, can be over-stimulating to the digestive system unless tempered by other colours, such as blues and greens. Red can heighten emotions and can cause recklessness and a lack of consideration, whereas warm shades of terracotta connect to the practical earthiness of cooking and baking.

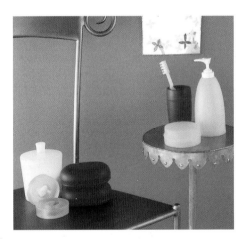

△ It is important to choose the appropriate shade of colour in decoration. A warm yellow in a kitchen is refreshing, a yellow that has more green in it may create the opposite effect.

◁ Bathrooms in bright, warm colours are enlivening and uplifting – though might encourage too much dawdling in a large family.

▽ Blue and white are classic colours to use in a bathroom, and in a room where there is plenty of natural light will bring a sense of clean tidiness without overwhelming coldness.

Blues and white are cool and efficient. They are not the best main colours for a kitchen that is a social space as well as an area of food preparation, but their clean freshness together makes them ideal as a colour for plates and other crockery. Cool colours in both rooms could be enhanced by the addition of a strong third colour to offset them. A luxurious space can be created by adding gold or a rich green to a stark blue and white setting.

Modern design's trend for wide expanses of stainless steel in kitchens is practical in commercial premises but can give an empty, unemotional feel to a family room that should be warm and welcoming.

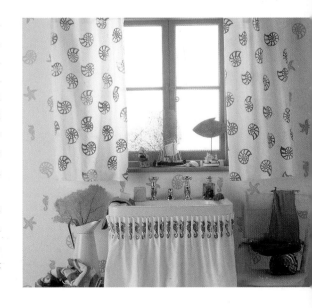

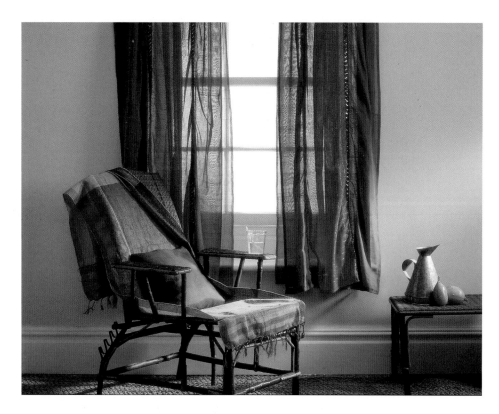

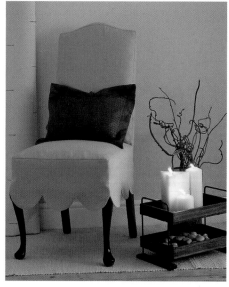

△ Brown promotes calm but this corner would benefit from a splash of yellow to add life.

△ This choice of colours will allow feelings of comfort, restfulness and a certain dreaminess to develop – ideal for a quiet space.

▽ Warm tones on large areas keep a space comfortable while spots of brighter colour bring individuality and visual interest.

living rooms

The only golden colour rule in the home is that if you dislike a particular colour – you should change it. Living in an atmosphere that you find disturbing in any way does not support health and wellbeing.

The main living area in the house needs to be a reflection of the owner's personality and should also be flexible enough to remain comfortable and generate a positive influence throughout all sorts of activities

▽ A collection of items with a range of complementary tones and hues creates a balance of energy, both visually and emotionally.

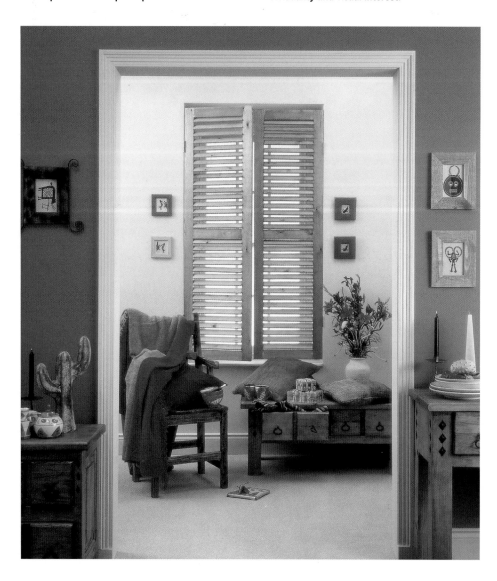

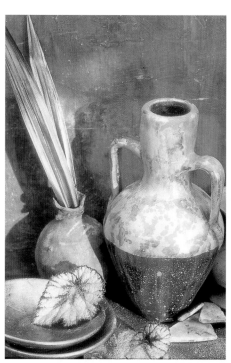

highlights of these colours will add depth and equilibrium to the home, maintaining a healthy balance of vibration.

Acquiring small items, such as cushions, throws or ornaments, that can be changed or their placement in the space rearranged, can be far more practical and flexible than adjusting large areas of colour in a room to reflect the energies of the people using it. Careful use of single coloured items can enhance a particular space. These items can be of similar tones or can be complementary colours for a subtle approach. Choosing contrasting colours can add a much more dramatic effect that draws attention to a particular area of the room.

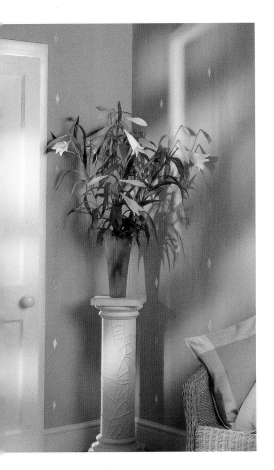

△ **Greens in nature display variation with the constant play of light. Indoors, greens are best in subtle, tempered shades.**

and moods. A background colour chosen from a pale version of one's favourite colour will be generally supportive and in harmony with the individual's energy field. If more than one person lives in a space a neutral tone can be chosen, or a compromise needs to be found so that everyone feels equally comfortable. For example, if one person's favourite colour is green and their partner's is blue, a turquoise colour scheme might be a good choice. Or, a complementary colour could be chosen, in this case a peach, gold or a pink tone.

Many people's choice of colours follows a similar pattern to other preferences in life. We prefer certain types of music and food, for example, but few of us would be happy just eating one thing all the time or listening endlessly to one piece of music. The same is true with colour. You may prefer tones that are within the turquoise through light blue to violet range of the spectrum, sometimes tending towards turquoise, other times towards magenta. If so, it is less likely that a yellow or red would appear in your colour scheme, but nonetheless, a few

INSTANT COLOUR

Keeping the main colour in the living area neutral means that it is a lot easier to change your surroundings from a cool, calm environment to a rich vibrant one, simply by swapping fabrics and soft furnishings. Add to this an adjustment in lighting, or even the addition of a few candles, and you have a cost-effective way of adjusting the overall ambience to suit your needs.

▽ **Even though complementary colours from the artist's colour wheel are used here, the red by its very nature is more dominant, bringing energy into a neutral white area.**

▽ **Blues with a hint of pink or violet have the quality of a warm summer sky and are inviting rather than isolating. A vase of vibrant orange flowers adds to the warmth.**

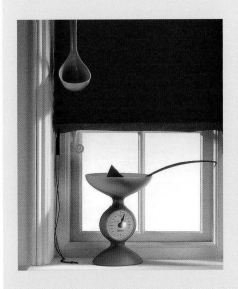

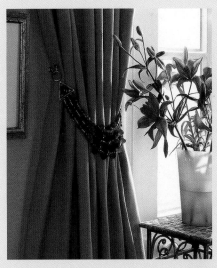

▽ **A calm blue background can be quickly enlivened with temporary elements if you are in need of some stimulation and energy.**

▽ **Chair covers that can be changed allow you to alter the feel of a space to suit your preferences at different times.**

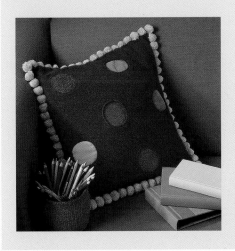

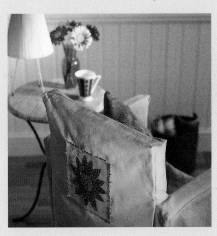

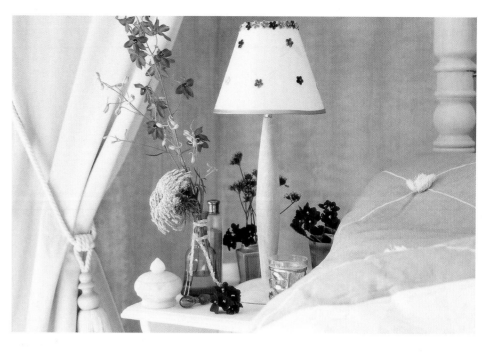

bedrooms

Perhaps the most important room in the house for most people is the bedroom, as this is where we spend the longest periods of time. These rooms are also our most individual and personal spaces so we need to be as comfortable in them as possible. Even a favourite colour can become a depressing influence if there is not a balance with other colours.

▽ Cool colours in a bedroom are perfect as they encourage the mind to quieten down and release the hectic activities of the day.

△ Blues and whites, especially with a hint of violet or purple are quietening, restful colours that help the body's natural sleep rhythms.

Colour favourites can also change quite quickly, especially with a greater awareness of the energy of colour vibrations. Generally speaking, colours that are restful and calming are better in bedrooms. Remember that the colour on the walls and fabrics will be having some effect on your energies even when you have your eyes shut. Muted and mixed tones are probably preferable to strong, bold colours. Blues calm the mind and lower the body's levels of activity, naturally encouraging sleep. Yellows, on the other hand, may be overstimulating – fine for waking up in the morning but not so good for getting a good night's rest. Pale violets will encourage relaxing, dreamy states and pale pinks will give a feeling of security.

▽ Pink and violet hues are light and calming and are good healing and recuperating colours.

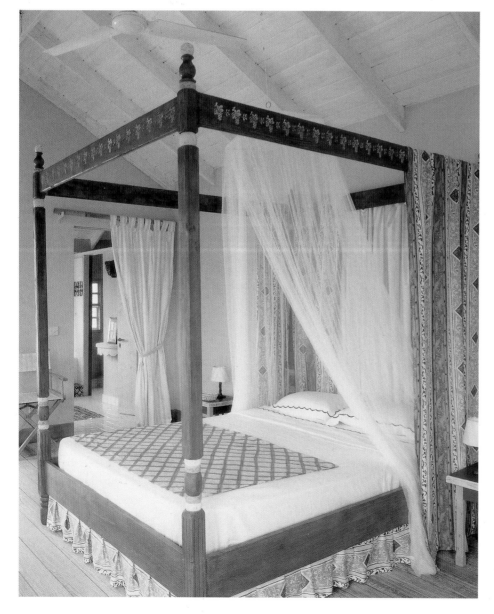

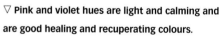

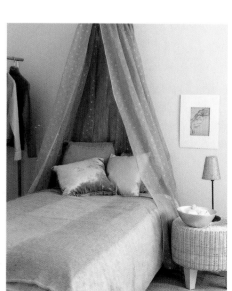

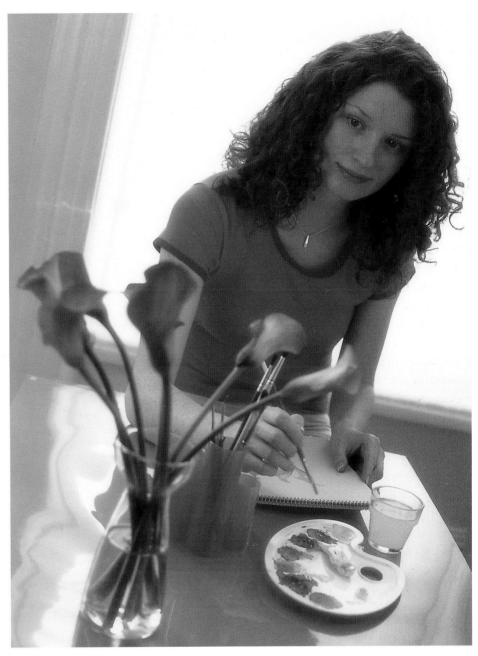

▷ Creative spaces are often made more effective when there is a range of colour energies – this encourages play but not necessarily mental focus.

▽ Restful expanses of colour can help mental focus for thinking and communicating.

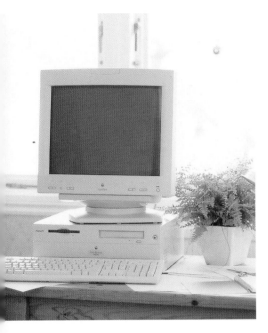

studies and workrooms

Work rooms such as studies and offices should reflect and complement the energy of the activity. Mental clarity and inspiration, for example, are promoted by bright yellow. and small amounts of yellow like a lampstand or letter rack, work just as well as yellow walls or curtains. Even a sheet of yellow card that can be placed in view can be very effective when you are feeling particularly tired. Cool blues are useful for calming down thought processes so that intuition and new ideas can emerge. In a busy space, where there is high energy and a fast pace, the presence of some blue can help to keep a peaceful ambience.

For physical dexterity and practical work, reds and oranges provide energy and focus, balanced by complementary greens to encourage calmness of mind and emotions. These colours are ideal combinations for sewing, painting and other creative arts, as they provide a comfortable space where work can be carried out for long periods.

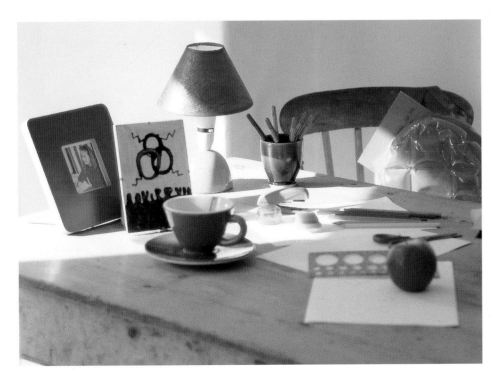

◁ Your own character will determine whether you work more effectively in an energizing or a sedating environment.

Feng Shui and colour

Feng shui (pronounced fung shoy) is a system that has developed to determine how we can live in a harmonious way with both our natural and man-made environments. It is a complex amalgamation of ideas and concepts from different sources.

A traditional feng shui assessment is taken from the whole site, from the building and from each room. People living in the house are taken into account, by looking at their personal astrological information. This traditional approach offers a complex assessment, and the results are often very different from the sparse interiors of some modern feng shui interpretations. A central theory of feng shui is that every object and colour possesses an energy that either enhances or detracts from the energy of those things around it. The purpose of feng shui is to balance all energy factors in a life supporting way.

feng shui basics

Across the world most cultures have evolved a philosophical model to unite the microcosm and the macrocosm, the inner with the outer, man with the world, earth with heaven. Heaven and earth are two fundamental polarities – the yin and yang of the Chinese system.

These polarities manifest themselves on earth as the four cardinal directions and the elements. Feng shui is based on the understanding of the movement and interaction of five fundamental types of energy – the elements. In the Chinese system these elements are described as wood, fire, earth, metal and water. The relationship of direction and element varies

▽ The principles of feng shui can blend with modern design to create a comfortable and harmonious space.

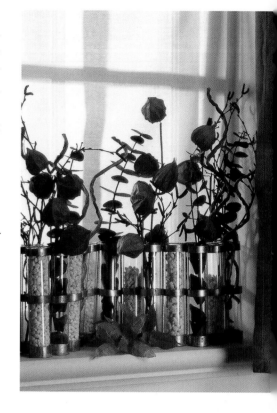

△ If the fire element needs balancing in the south of a space or if there is too much of the water element, red and orange objects can help.

between cultures, as does the number of elements and their description. Most divisions have earth, air, fire and water with space or ether being the fifth.

Feng shui developed from a shamanic assessment of the energies in a landscape so that human activities and buildings would not interfere with the natural flow of ch'i or life-force. Over the centuries it gathered ideas from Taoism, Bön (Tibet's shamanic tradition) and Buddhism as well as folk magic. It can be a deeply philosophical understanding of how cosmic energy moves through the world, or it can appear to be talismanic magic, offering quick fixes to every problem in life.

how to implement feng shui

Colour is one of the nine basic cures of feng shui. Because each element is assigned a colour (see elements box) it is possible to

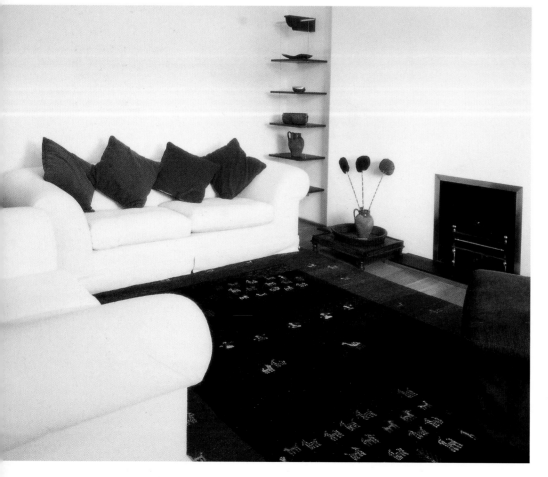

THE ELEMENTS

The main energies that a feng shui practitioner needs to balance.

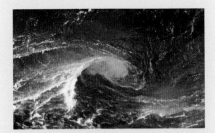

△ The element of water is linked to the north, blue and black.

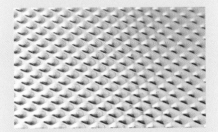

△ The element of metal is linked to the west, white and silver.

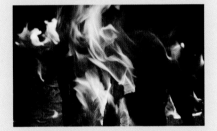

△ The element of fire is linked to the south and the colour red.

△ The element of earth is the centre and is yellow.

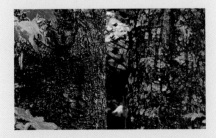

△ The element of wood is linked to the east, green and blue.

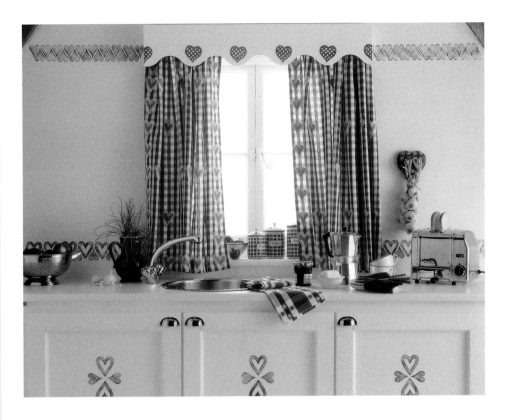

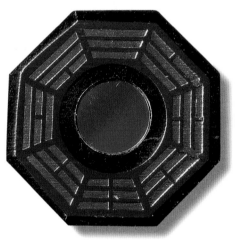

△ The pa kua represents all the elements and directions. With a central mirror for removing stagnant energy it is a vital feng shui cure.

△ If the sink is located in the northern quarter of the kitchen, using red near it may help to balance out an over-emphasis on the water element.

balance an environment by placing objects of the appropriate colour in the correct direction. Every factor of direction, shape, material and relationship needs to be taken into account to balance a space according to feng shui, but introducing some colours that reflect the elements can be a simple way of establishing a harmonious relationship within the environment.

Following the Five Element system of feng shui, the north is associated with blue and black and its element is water. The east is associated with green and blue and its element is wood. The south is associated with red and its element is fire. The west is associated with white and silver and its element is metal. At the centre is yellow, representing the earth.

If you are unable to make large changes to the colours in a room by painting walls or altering fabrics, you can make symbolic adjustments with ornaments representing the elements or directions. For example, a bright red object or piece of fabric will introduce the fire element, while a representation of a fish or a sea shell will bring in the water element.

▽ Simply placing appropriately coloured objects in each elemental area can restore balance.

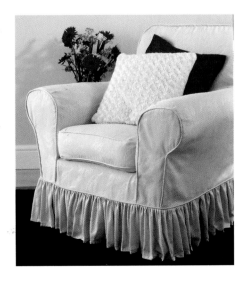

The Colour Palette

Each colour has a set of clearly defined influences and meanings, which can be invaluable in understanding the world around us and our behaviour patterns. These qualities can also be used to create particular impressions on others. A desired image or a subtle message can be sent with colour much more effectively than with words.

Red

Red is the colour with the longest wavelength. It is the nearest visible light to infrared in the electromagnetic spectrum. Although red occurs beyond the infrared, it maintains close connections with heat and warmth. Even rocks will become red when they are heated sufficiently. This is seen in volcanic eruptions when lava pours out on to the surface of the earth.

living red

Instinctively, the occurrence of red makes us wary, as we connect it with heat and the potential danger of burning. Red lights are

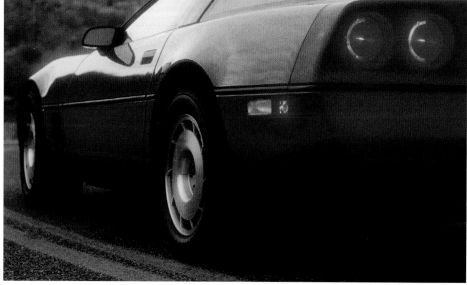

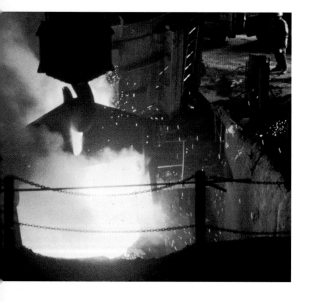

△ **Red is the colour of heat and burning. Infrared is invisible to the human eye but its heating effects are evident when hot objects appear red.**

▽ **The effect of red on the eye is quite unusual. For the colour to be seen, the eye itself makes internal adjustments. This alteration means that we see red objects as closer than they really are.**

built into artificial fires to help simulate the cosiness of a real fire. Too much heat and red burns, but at the right level it supports our lives and gives us comfort.

Being the colour of blood, red has symbolic links with living and life. Spilling or losing blood brings illness and death. Wearing red, eating red foods and surrounding yourself with red increases the body's ability to absorb iron, the metal that is responsible for the colour of haemoglobin in the blood. The presence of haemoglobin allows the blood to absorb oxygen in the lungs and to transport that life-giving oxygen to the cells of the body.

Physical activity and the energy that supports it also has a red vibration. If speed, danger, daring or courage are involved, the red quality of the activity increases. Mountaineers, racing car drivers and stuntmen all have 'red' careers.

feeling red

Phrases like 'red light district' and 'scarlet woman' aptly describe the sexual nature of red. Some aspects of red behaviour are not socially acceptable. Red together with black is associated with evil, for example in the archetypal 'red devil' of medieval artists.

△ **The cliché of what the red sports car is thought to represent sums up the dynamic, direct, self-absorbed quality of red energy.**

PUT RED IN YOUR LIFE WHEN THERE IS ...

• a lack of enthusiasm and interest in life
• a lack of energy and a feeling of over-tiredness
• an inability to make your dreams a practical reality
• a feeling of insecurity, unwarranted fear, or anxiety

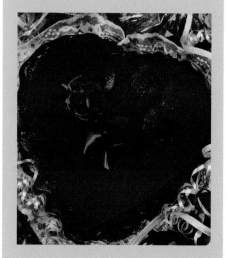

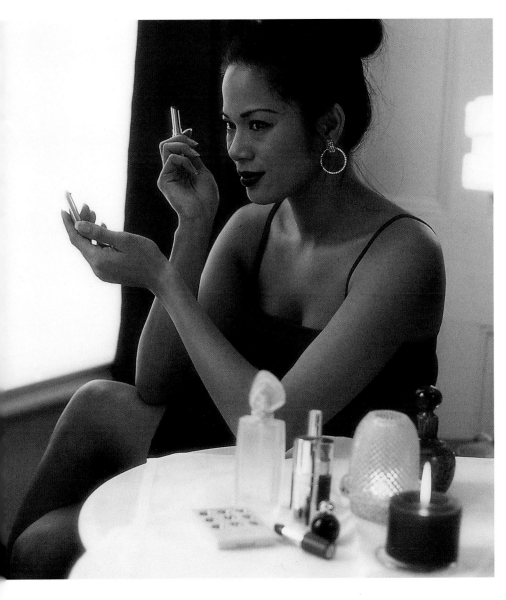

△ When a woman wears the colour red, it has an immediacy and boldness. It says 'I am here, notice me' and is closely associated with sex appeal, and also with illicit passion.

who abuse it. These people often display some of the negative qualities that are associated with red – selfishness and an interest only in personal, rather than global, survival and short-term security.

To be healthy in a long-term sense, we need the colour red to reconnect ourselves to the planet and support it as it supports us. For our personal development, the role involves taking responsibility for our own wellbeing and survival as part of humanity as a whole, not being separate from it. Although often seen as a 'green' issue, global and local conservation is also about survival, which is a red issue. Red and green issues are intrinsically linked, as they are complementary colours.

Blatant expression of emotion is not always easy to handle, whether it is sexuality, passion, anger or aggression. When expressing red emotions, the heart beats faster, the capillaries dilate and the skin becomes flushed and feels warm.

Red is thought of as an immediate colour. This affects the thinking processes, causing restlessness and impatience. Red can result in very selfish behaviour, a focus on personal needs and survival above everything else. Sometimes the drive to survive is what fuels

△ Red can easily lead to excess as its own nature is impulsive and reckless. Drunken behaviour exemplifies many qualities of too much red energy.

impulsive actions and rash comments. When these traits are managed well they create capable business people who are innovators and entrepreneurs, preferring to move from one project to another, getting an operation on its feet then moving on. They are gifted with being able to manifest new ideas. Often people with red traits are also renowned for their daring exploits, and they can be somewhat extrovert and boastful about their skills.

Red brings focus to the physicality of life, to the process of living. The colour is symbolic of what we need to survive. Life should be grabbed and lived with a sense of immediacy. Without red we become listless and out of touch with reality and we fail to live our dreams in this world. Without the foundation that red gives us we just daydream of escaping into fantasty worlds.

Red keeps us rooted in the red energy of our planet. People who become detached or divorced from the planet tend to be those

USING RED

If you want to come across as a bold and dynamic person, wear a red scarf or a tie. This is especially effective if you have an event coming up at which your confidence needs a boost, such as an interview or a presentation. You might also find this useful for a social occasion when you feel nervous about some new people.

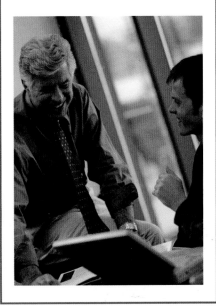

Orange

While red is associated with fiery heat, orange is more closely linked to the benign warmth of the sun and of fire. Like fire, orange energy displays some sense of direction and purpose – it moves along those pathways which fuel its own existence. Orange is certainly dynamic, but more thoughtful and controlled than explosive red. As a mixture of red and yellow, orange blends the properties of both primary colours. (The secondary colours – orange, green and violet – are also able to balance contrasting energies.) Curiosity is one of the driving characteristics of the orange vibration and this brings exploration and creativity, particularly on a practical level.

PUT ORANGE IN YOUR LIFE WHEN THERE IS ...

• a feeling of bleakness and boredom, particularly where there is a sense that time is really dragging
• a lack of interest in what is going on around you, even to the degree of disdaining to become involved in any way
• a resentment of changes in familiar routines and an obsessive need to have things in their 'proper' place
• over-seriousness – taking oneself too seriously, being unable to see humour and playfulness in life
• a fear of experiencing pleasure through the senses and of enjoying sensuality
• an inability to let go of the past. This can be especially apparent after an accident or shock where the mind continually revolves around the issues involved – the 'what if ...' and 'if only I had done this instead of that ...'
• a problem with blocked experiences in life, such as a decrease in personal creativity

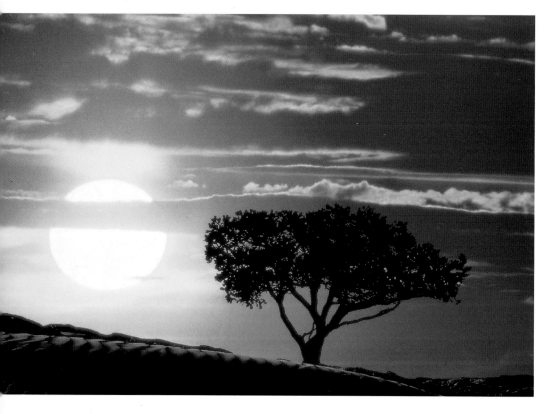

△ Orange warms without burning. The light of sunrise and sunset encourages a sensitivity to creative ideas and contemplative thought.

▷ A fox cub illustrates how orange promotes exploration, play and creativity.

▽ Orange combines the new energy of red with the organizing qualities of yellow.

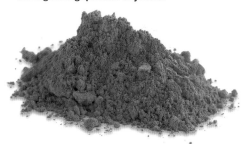

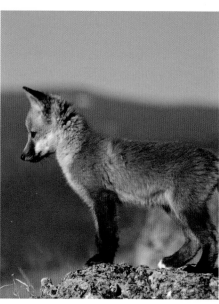

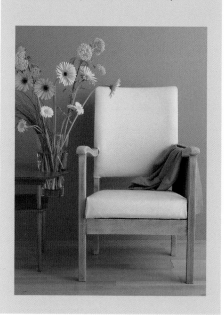

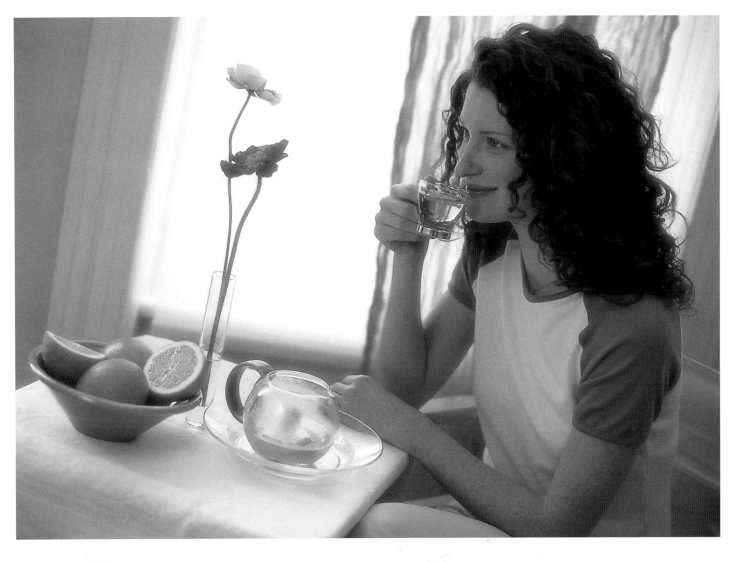

playing at life

While red is a focusing or self-centred energy, orange reaches out to see what it feels like to be somewhere else – it is the toddler trying to grasp and wanting to taste everything. Orange is learning to experience the world with a sense of play and enjoyment.

Strangely, surveys have often found orange to be the least popular of colours (the favourites being green and blue). Exploring and reaching out can sometimes be painful. We learn that stroking a cat's fur is enjoyable and fun, but pulling a cat's whiskers can lead to the pain of a swift retaliation. Learning by exploring is somewhat risky, full of unknowns – this is the element of excitment, but it can also bring shock and stress. Yet because the orange energy is purposeful and has an instinct for moving on, it can creatively remove blocks to restriction and stagnation.

Orange represents instinctive rather than intellectual or thought-out problem solving. Orange energy often manifests itself

△ **Orange peel – washed first, or from organic sources – makes a soothing tea that aids digestion and helps to relax the body and release any feelings of stress.**

when someone is working on the design of their garden. It can also emerge through a potter working clay, or an artist roughing out a sketch, or a poet scribbling ideas. Even doodling on a pad while listening to someone on the telephone is exhibiting the natural urge to explore through creativity – to allow a flow of energy to balance the sense of identity characterised by red.

A balance of orange energy brings a willingness to get involved, to 'get one's hands dirty' with practical exploration. It gives the ability to fill time creatively and to be aware of the needs of the body. Without orange energy, attention tends to get drawn to the head, filling our lives with ideas, thoughts and theories. Orange enables us to put these thought processes into practice in the world in a creative way, and to enjoy the experience of doing so.

USING ORANGE
In times of stress, or after a shock or a surprise, wearing shades of orange can help the body to return to a state of balance.

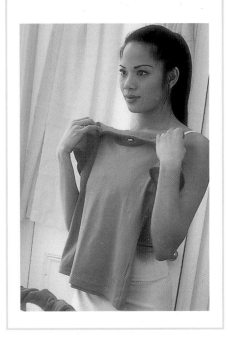

Yellow

Yellow is a bright, sunny colour. Most people will recognize the sensation of warmth and vitality when looking at a strong, pure yellow. Like the energy of a bright, sunny morning yellow brings clarity and awareness. As with all colours, different yellows will create markedly different responses. An orange-yellow or golden colour imparts a sense of establishment, of solidity and assuredness, a rich, round sensation of inner warmth. A clean, light yellow seems to clear the mind while keeping it alert and active

PUT YELLOW IN YOUR LIFE WHEN THERE IS ...

- confusion and indecision
- fear and anxiety caused by unknown factors leading to nervous and digestive disorders
- a weak and confused immune system – frequent minor illnesses, intolerances and allergies to foods and other substances
- nervous exhaustion, nervous breakdown, 'burn out', panic attacks, hot flushes
- poor memory, inability to concentrate or study
- tendency to Seasonal Affective Disorder (SAD) or lethargy and depression in dull weather
- digestive difficulties, malabsorption of food

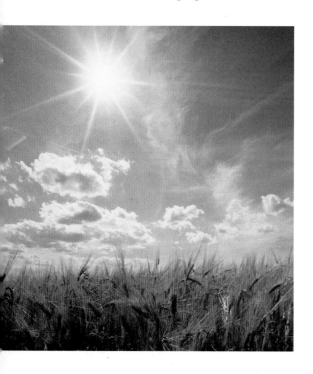

△ **The light of the morning sun is stimulating and enlivening to plants and daytime creatures.**

▽ **Yellow enriches, lightens and activates many of the systems of the body. It tends to encourage orderliness and clarity.**

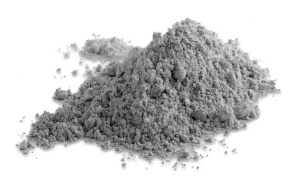

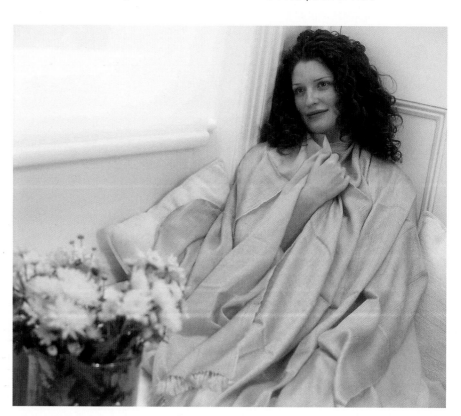

in a state of readiness. An acid yellow can be stimulating and enlivening, a shade of yellow that has just a touch of green, however, will create a degree of discomfort, disorientation and even nausea.

decisive yellow

The functions of the yellow vibration have to do with decision-making, with what to do in any given situation. Decisions rely on information, but more importantly on the ability to select bits of information that are relevant. Discrimination, knowing what is what, is a 'yellow' skill upon which we constantly rely for our wellbeing, physically as well as mentally.

The digestive system, the immune system and the nervous system all reflect yellow frequencies. The functions of the digestive system are to break down, identify and absorb those substances that the body requires for maintenance and growth, and to eliminate from the system those substances that are harmful or unnecessary. The

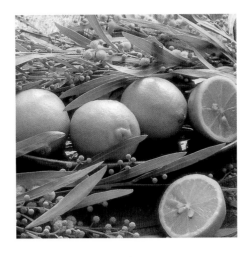

▷ The colour yellow is naturally associated with the sun itself, and so with its life-giving and sustaining energies. Lemons and yellow flowers are instant reminders of these qualities and an easy way to access them.

▽ Honey, the concentrated energy of sunlight turned into nectar sugars by plants and processed by bees, has many yellow qualities: it helps the digestive system, is gently energizing and is a powerful immune system booster.

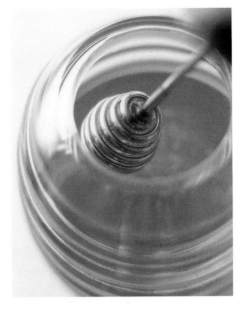

immune system works in a similar way. Its various organs and defences are able to identify and destroy cells that are in the wrong place or have come into the body from outside, such as bacteria and viruses.

The digestive system and the immune system rely on correct decisions about what is useful and what is dangerous. Both need qualities of intelligence, memory and discrimination. If for some reason, such as stress, the systems fail to work as well as they should, mistakes are made: the digestion may not absorb nutrients that are needed and the immune system may identify harmless substances as dangerous, creating intolerance or allergic reactions.

The nervous system relays information to the brain, which then categorizes, interprets and acts upon the signals. Correct identification of priorities leads to an easy relationship with the world. When this yellow function is lacking, confusion and indecision creep in. Fear and worry are the consequence of an imbalance of yellow energy, when wrong information and a lack of clear and logical thought result in an inability to act positively.

Society in the West is currently very focused on the yellow qualities of acquisition of knowledge, organization, structure and information exchange. The senses are continually bombarded with information, and large amounts of yellow energy are used up. However, people in this work environment spend the day in artificial light and are badly lacking in the yellow energy of sunlight. As a result, they need additional yellow from food, furnishings and sunlight to help keep the balance in their busy lives.

USING YELLOW

When working at a computer use a yellow mouse mat to improve your concentration and stay alert.

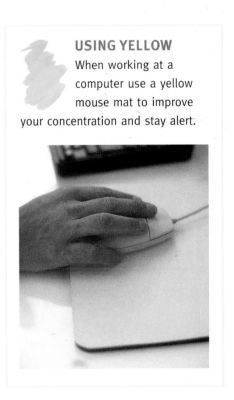

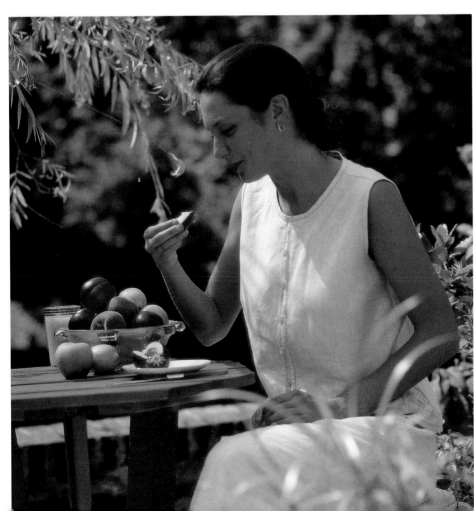

◁ Eating outside in natural sunlight improves digestion and gives a feeling of wellbeing.

Green

Green is the colour of nature, the colour of the plant kingdoms. The human eye has its greatest sensitivity in the range of frequencies we perceive as green. Perhaps this skill evolved during mankind's early development as a forest dweller. The qualities of green are characterized by balance, and indeed green itself is found midway in the spectrum. Whereas the reds and yellows are warm colours, and the blues and violets are cool, green can be seen as either, depending on the shade.

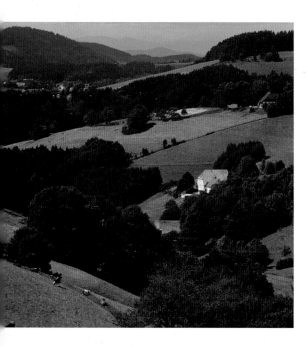

△ **Personal space and a sense of freedom helps to relax emotional and physical tensions. We respond to such views by taking a deep breath.**

▽ **The human eye recognizes more variation of colour in green than in any other colour. Individual choice can therefore be very particular.**

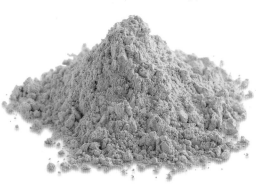

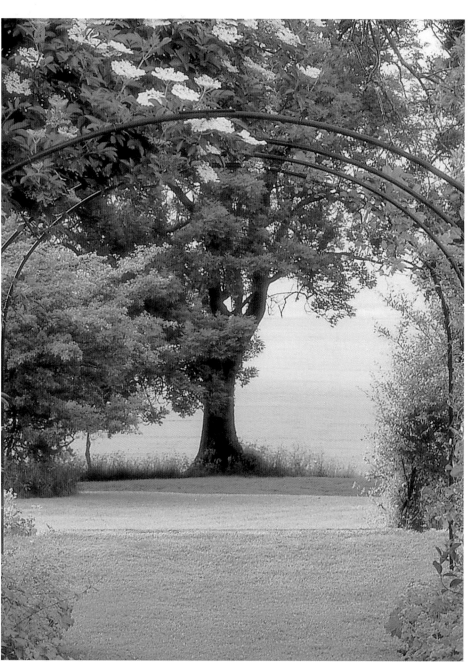

green growth

The power of nature is green power. Green stands for growth and the desire to expand and increase. Yet growth requires change, and change means that what has been must disappear to be replaced by what is to come. The process of life is the process of transformation from one state to another, the death of one form giving birth to another. Balance and a sense of order must be present for growth. Growth is an expansion of

△ **The need to expand, grow and increase is a core quality of green energy expressed in nature.**

orderliness that must be sustainable, with each stage acting as a foundation for the next period of expansion.

green relationships

The colour green is the vibration of relationships, because in growing and expanding we meet others in the world around us.

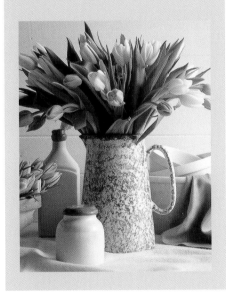

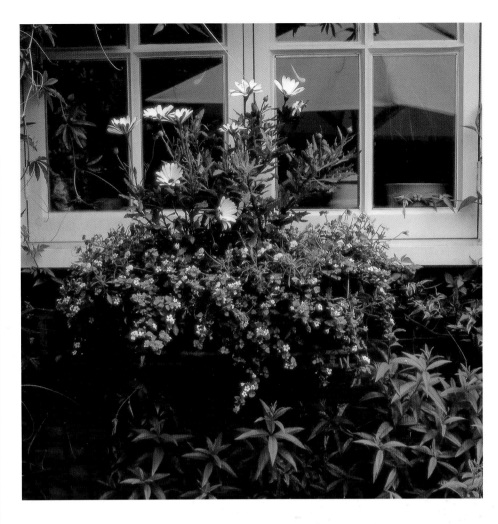

△ For people who work and live away from a natural environment, gardens and urban parks help to restore balance and perspective. Even a simple window box can have this effect.

Learning how to relate to others is a skill of balancing our needs with the needs of the other person. If it is possible to develop a mutually agreeable relationship of caring and sharing, both lives are enriched and expanded – our interaction with the world is broadened. When a relationship is formed that is negative, manipulative or unpleasant in some way – very often because one person is trying to gain power and control over the other (a negative green tendency) – then our own potential for understanding the world is curtailed and restricted.

Green energy inevitably has to do with the pushing out of boundaries, of growing beyond what is known. Because it is expansive it must develop relationships with those things around it, but it must also have a degree of power and control.

The power of green can be expressed in a harmonious way, as in an ecological balance where all elements are accommodated and mutually supportive, or it can be destructive to everything around it, simply absorbing or taking over, enforcing new order on others. The energy that green creates is the energy of finding direction and new paths. Green enables us to find the means to the desired end; it provides the power to accomplish rather than power to dominate. In this way green shows how to balance difficult extremes to enable progress to be made.

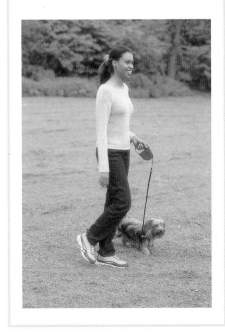

Blue

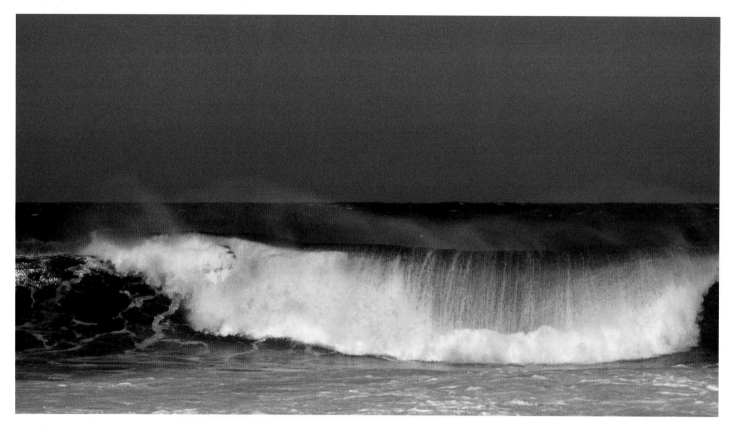

Blue is the colour of distance. When artists of the early Renaissance began to consider how to represent perspective, they employed the simple observation that in nature the further away an object was in space, the more blue it appeared. When we think of blue in this way it is associated with looking beyond what is in the immediate environment – and the colour itself also has the effect of stretching the perceptions outwards to the unknown.

▽ **The peaceful, restful energy of blue has almost universal popularity, and imbues the qualities of steadiness and reliability.**

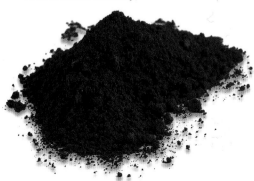

△ **The blues that are found in the sea and sky help to free the mind from its normal activity.**

communicative blue

There are two aspects of blue. On the one hand there is the experience of going beyond what is known – the active search for information or detail – and on the other hand the experience of rest and peacefulness, simply being happy to be alive without any particular focus of thought.

In some respects these seem to be contradictory qualities but in fact the uniting factor is the desire for equilibrium. For example, the teacher is better informed than the student. Communication allows the student to learn what the teacher knows. The teaching will stop when the teacher and student know the same information. This is a new state of equilibrium and peace that will continue until a new source of information is found and interaction begins again. All kinds of communication, like talking, listening, learning and the exchange

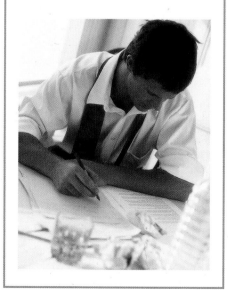

USING BLUE
Blue will help the easy flow of communication whether it is with other people or listening to your own thoughts and feelings. To help remember a speech, write your notes on blue paper.

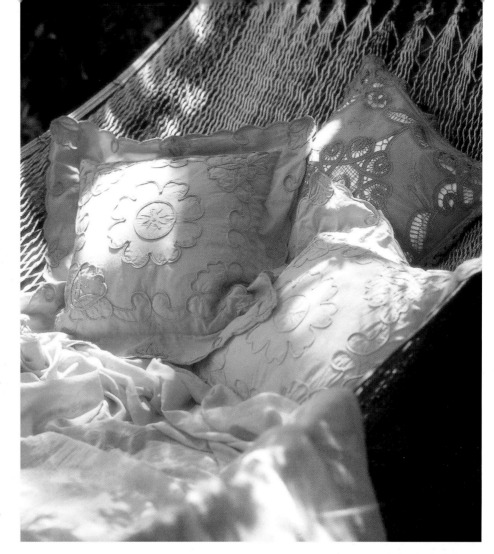

▷ Using the colour blue in a situation of relaxation and repose will encourage quiet communication and feelings of peace.

of information and viewpoints are blue activities. So too, are the expressive arts – not just the performing arts such as acting, singing and music, but any art form that seeks to communicate with other people. Any of the five senses can be used to tell the story or carry the message.

Although blue is the colour of communication and the flow of energy it is a cool vibration. We can understand this property when we consider that redness or heat is often caused by a concentration or build-up of energy that cannot flow freely. Thus inflammation – a red, energetic state – in the body can be reduced by cooling the area down by using a blue vibration. This will counteract the red quality, or will help to remove the block and to create a flow of energy, thus enabling the area to return to normal functioning.

▽ Blue encourages an effective flow of peace and understanding. Many compassionate deities are associated with blue. The robes of the Virgin Mary are predominantly blue indicating her ability to hear and respond to humanity.

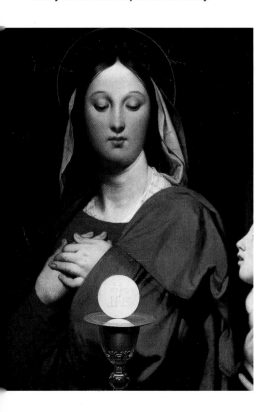

distant emotions

The sense of distance gives blue a quality of detachment and devotion. Gazing into the sky naturally brings a sense of peace. The colour blue somehow seems to free the mind from its normal activity, removing us slightly from involvement with thought, emotion or physical action. A 'cool' personality avoids getting caught up in emotional turmoil or any particular belief. That impersonal quality is like the blue of the distant mountains, not overwhelmed by detail or closeness, but offering the possibility of greater perspectives. Blue is also linked to devotion. This is the quality of the vibration that can be understood as a constant stream of energy or communication towards the source of devotion, which is usually a powerful, universal focus of great depth such as the Virgin Mary, Krishna or Shiva – all of whom are associated with the colour blue.

Without some injection of blue in our lives helping the flow of information and energy, we will inevitably experience frustration, disappointment and lack of progress in whatever we do.

PUT BLUE IN YOUR LIFE WHEN THERE IS ...
- a need to calm agitated, excitable, or chaotic states
- a need to communicate clearly
- a need for help with new information or in seeing information in context
- a need for peace, detachment, solitude and rest

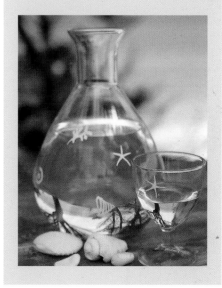

Indigo

There is a different quality to the experience of looking at a cloudless blue sky and a midnight blue sky. The indigo of the midnight sky amplifies the characteristics of blue in a profound, resonant way. At a physical level, while blue is a quietening and cooling colour, indigo is sedating. In a depressed state indigo is to be avoided as it can easily deepen the mood.

how indigo works

In a way, indigo turns blue energy inwards: while blue promotes some form of communication between people, indigo creates an internal communication in an individual that might manifest as profound thought processes, new insights, philosophy and

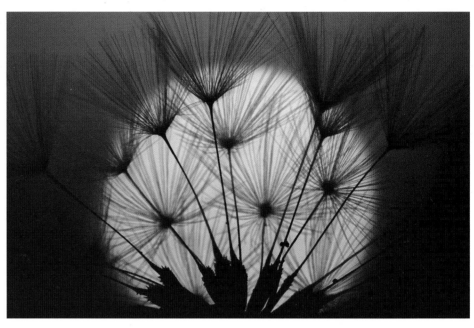

△ **The midnight sky has an infinite depth that reflects the timeless quality of indigo light.**

intuition. The flow of blue can be fast, but the flow of indigo can be almost instantaneous, often leading to the sensation of inspiration 'coming out of the blue', with no previous development or build-up of thoughts and ideas. Intuition and sudden clarity of awareness, startling realizations and innovative concepts occur in the 'super-cooled' state of indigo.

The depths of indigo may seem unfathomable and mysterious, but they can yield useful perceptions. Indigo is related to clairvoyance, clairsentience and clairaudience (clear seeing, feeling and hearing) and other psychic skills.

▽ **Indigo pigment was derived from azurite and lapis lazuli and was an expensive commodity. Woad is one of the few vegetable dyes to produce the same deep blue colour.**

PUT INDIGO IN YOUR LIFE WHEN THERE IS ...

- a need to focus on personal issues, beliefs and ideas
- a need to develop sensitivity to the inner senses and intuition
- a need to cool and quieten normal mental processes
- a need to relieve physical, mental and emotional pain
- inability or difficulty in assimilating and understanding new concepts or philosophies
- a need for temporary relief and removal from everyday problems and difficult experiences in life
- a need for space and a desire for a period of solitude

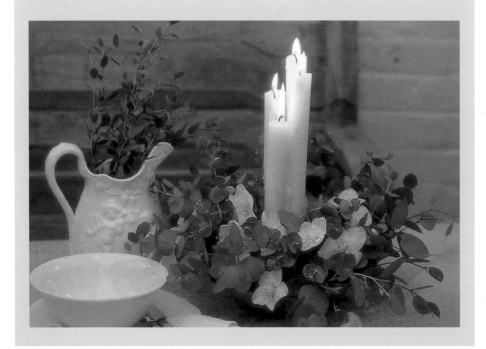

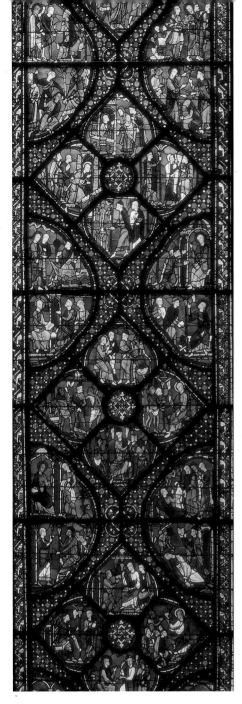

△ The wonderful stained glass windows of Chartres cathedral in France are a masterpiece of medieval design, bathing the interior with a deep blue light that heightens the sensitivities and elevates awareness from the mundane world.

▽ Blueberries and sloes are some of the indigo foods that can be found growing wild.

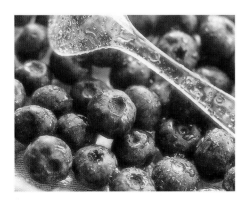

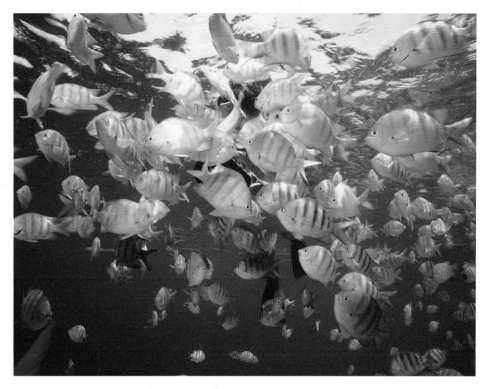

△ In an indigo state of awareness, the stillness of the mind is unperturbed by thoughts that come and go – like fish moving through deep water.

profound indigo

The deep, directionless depths of indigo can sedate the conscious mind to a degree where more subtle, delicate perceptions can be registered. Blue energy is the skill of language and eloquence personified in the talker. Indigo energy definitely belongs to the listener. Blue energy can be frivolous and superficial, but indigo energy never fails to be profound and significant.

The internal quality of indigo and the enhanced sense of removal from normal, everyday communication can mean that those using a lot of indigo energy are able to step away from how the world is usually seen and come up with new and startling ways of thinking. The inventor has these qualities, going beyond the consensus view of what is possible while often appearing to be socially out of step or isolated. The internalizing qualities of indigo make it an ideal colour to use in contemplative and spiritual contexts, particularly in solitary meditations, and in visualization, where the inner senses are given a higher importance than the physical senses. Without the qualities provided by indigo we would need to find other resources to help provide deep quiet in our lives.

USING INDIGO
To find peace for reflection, look up at the clear night sky. Contemplation and deep meditation come easier in the indigo depths of night. Night-time is often when inspirations and solutions to problems naturally arise.

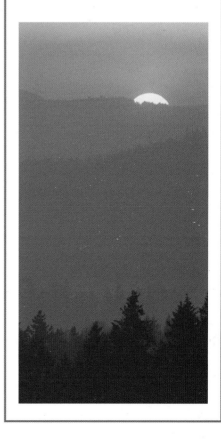

Violet

Violet is the colour at the opposite end of the rainbow spectrum to red. A combination of blue and red, it can be seen both as a completion and as the beginning of another cycle of vibratory energy, the rest of which ascends beyond the visible spectrum. Violet is the door to the unseen, both in terms of the electromagnetic spectrum and in human experience.

how violet works

The key to understanding the energy of violet is to see how its component colours work together.

Red is a focusing, concentrating, dynamic and activating energy, while blue is a cooling, quietening and expansive energy. Violet brings a new dynamism to the unfocused expansion of blue and a stabilizing energy to the frenetic activity of red. The rather undirected spaciousness of blue is made practical by the addition of

◁ **Aubergines (eggplant) are part of the *solanacea* family which also includes deadly nightshade and tobacco, and contain toxic alkaloids, which can distort our perception of reality, a very violet characteristic.**

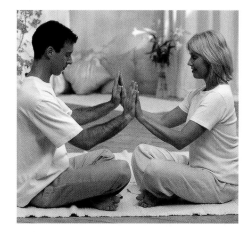

△ **Healing is represented by the colour violet – the blue giving detachment and the ability to be devoted to the flow of energy, and the red supplying motivation to be of use to others.**

the red. Concepts and ideas are thus better able to find some real application in the world. The energy that red brings allows more creative qualities to emerge from the blue, so violet is associated with the imagination and with inspiration.

violet and fantasy

The difficulty with the world of violet energy is that it can become very self-contained. The red and blue make such a balanced whole that it is easy not to look

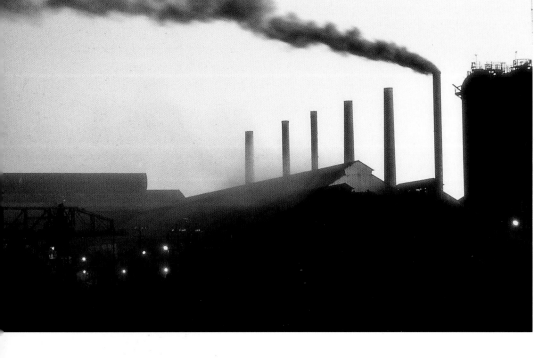

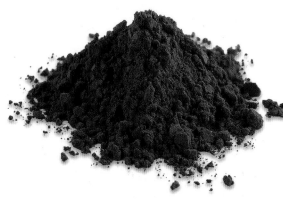

△ **The silhouette of an industrial landscape, beautifully etched on a violet sky, illustrates this colour's ability to combine and balance the practical with the ideal, dreams with reality.**

◁ **Violet energy ranges from blue with a hint of red, to purple, where the red and blue are more equally mixed.**

▷ **Quiet, meditative spaces can benefit from a touch of violet colour.**

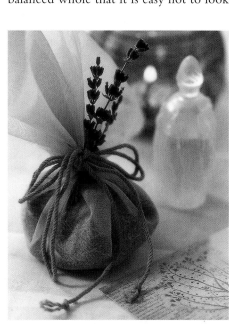

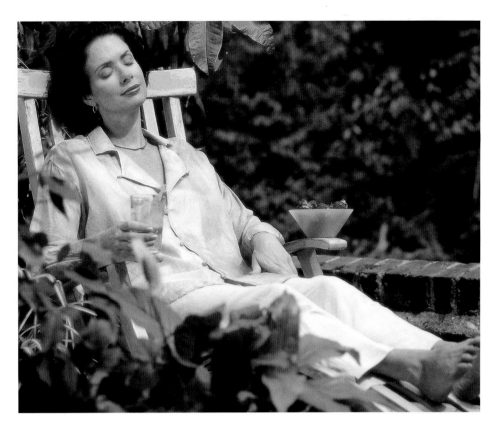

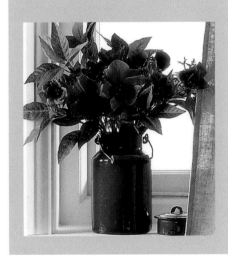

beyond it. Where this happens, imagination transforms into fantasy, and inspiration becomes fanaticism. Violet energy, because it seems to extend beyond our current knowledge into the unknown, can trap the spiritual dreamer in a fantastic world of miraculous happenings and unrealistic wishful thinking. Here the practical world and all its tangible solidity is rejected in favour of a make-believe, usually very selfish, sense of personal evolution or spiritual progress.

▷ **Violet and purple suggest
luxury, even today, a lasting
memory of the time
when these colours
were exclusive to
the rich.**

△ **Violet encourages the flow of the imagination
and the integration of ideas, or it can degenerate
into daydreams and fantasy.**

If the lure of the glamorous unknown can be avoided, violet energy can become one of the most effective colours to bring balance and healing in any situation. It helps to integrate energies at every level and as healing requires the building up of new systems (red energy), according to accurate information (blue energy), violet can speed both physical and emotional recovery.

Violet is an important energy to those who use the blue and indigo skills of psychic perception, because it helps to supply the grounding energy for the work. Without the anchoring abilities of red, the use of subtle perceptions can seriously imbalance and exhaust the life-energy of the practitioner.

The skill of integration is aided by violet. As the colour combines opposite energies, it can help people who need to work with an array of disparate things. Violet is often associated with the richness and diversity of ceremony, perhaps originating from its ability to psychologically balance the minds

and actions of the participants. Violet is often thought to be the most spiritual of all colours. In bygone days, violet dye was expensive and reserved for the priesthood and the rich. In practice, though, no colour is more spiritual than any other.

USING VIOLET
Lavender is a traditional remedy for insomnia or restlessness at night. It is also one of the most versatile essential oils for scratches, burns, headaches and worry. Dried lavender flowers beside the bed, or a drop of oil on the pillow, will encourage peaceful sleep.

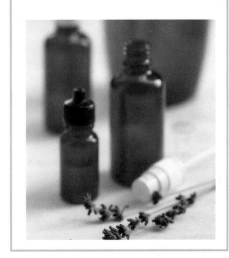

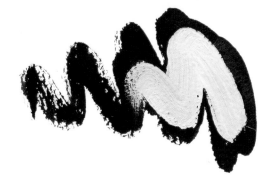

White and black

When people speak of opposites it is usually in terms of black and white. Strictly speaking neither are colours – simply characteristics of the presence or absence of light. As in all polarities, black and white cannot be defined without each other. Like day and night, white and black are part of an unceasing definition of existence.

white absolutes

The presence of white is what humans perceive as the entire visible light spectrum seen

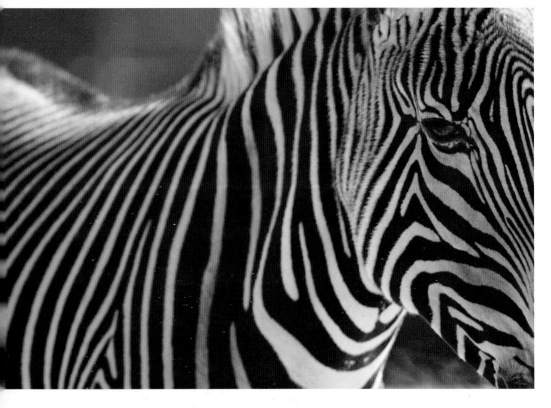

▷ Coal and soot consist of black carbon – one of the earliest used pigments.

together – the complete energy of light. In this sense it stands for wholeness and completion – nothing has been taken out, everything is present. In many cultures white is associated with purity and cleanliness, openness and truth – everything is shown in bright light, nothing is hidden. This is why white is often used to denote holiness. White is also the colour of bone and the snow of winter, so for some, the energy of white relates to the starkness of death and endings. Both of these interpretations, purity and death, are connected by the act of

USING BLACK
If you want to become inconspicuous, consider dressing in black. Black can be inconspicuous, or it can make a bold statement of mystery and self-control. Black clothes often say; 'notice my presence but don't intrude into my space'.

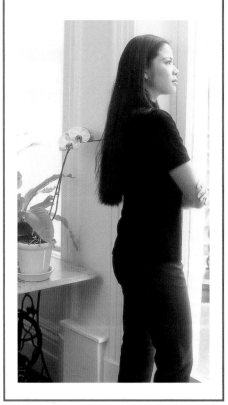

setting things apart from normal life, creating a sense of specialness. Entering or leaving the world, white signifies beginnings and the end of one cycle that enables another to start.

White is uncompromising. Everything is clear, open and explicitly manifest. It has a cold quality. White can be of use when clarity is needed in life. But it can also take on a hint of the other colours around it and so acts like a mirror to the energies that are in proximity. This can make it a rather uncomfortable colour for those who do not wish to have their hidden feelings reflected

△ Light and shade, black and white, the zebra takes advantage of random contrasting patterns to disappear into its surroundings.

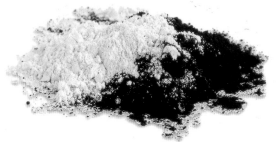

◁ Black and white are associated with viewpoints where no mutual ground can be found yet neither can exist without the other.

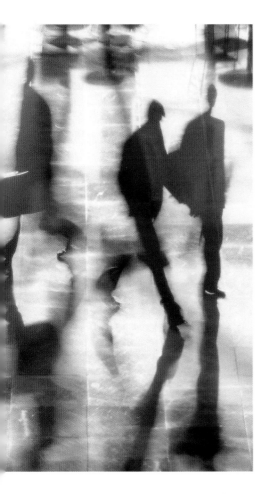

△ **Where there is light and three-dimensional form there is shadow, each defines the other.**

back to them. As a vibration of purification, white can help to clarify all aspects of life, giving the energy to sweep away blocks in physical, emotional and mental patterns. There are no degrees of white, and its action can be as uncompromising and rapid as a flash of blinding light. White gives the potential to move towards every other colour, as it allows development in any direction. It is a good choice for new beginnings.

black contrasts

White reflects all aspects of light, but black absorbs all aspects of light. So while white reveals, black conceals. In the simplicity of symbolism white is translated as whole, holy and good, so black inevitably becomes linked to the hidden, fearful and bad experiences. Black is the fear of a starless, moonless night where everything is unseen and unknown and anything might be hiding out there to wish us harm. Where white is the colour of emergence, of birth and change, black is the colour of continuity, of withdrawal from definition, of the hidden. White continually makes its presence felt:

it shouts 'I am here!' Black withdraws, refusing to take a stand or be noticed. White is the energy of completion, an expanse outwards. Black is the energy of gestation and of preparation. Black has often been associated with the energies of the earth and the fertile soil. The rich earth from which all life and sustenance springs is the same earth where the dead are placed.

In a way, both white and black reflect the particular beliefs of the individual. White can be seen negatively as blankness, and positively as a clean slate, offering a new beginning. In times of fear and uncertainty, black is a threatening unknown, a silence in which our own terrors and nightmares can be amplified. But at other times, black may simply be experienced as a restful emptiness that allows many different possibilities to emerge and disappear again.

▽ **Black can be seen as a threatening colour, representing a cloak over what lies beneath or within. At other times it is mysterious, allowing a sense of potential or possibility. It is the energy of gestation and preparation.**

USING WHITE
White has the ability to clear away all clutter, all extraneous noise. Fresh starts and new beginnings all benefit from its energy. Looking at a picture of snow-clad mountains brings clarity and freshness to a mind that feels crowded.

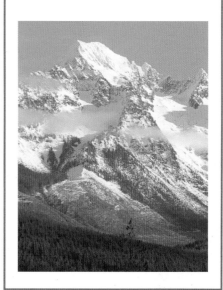

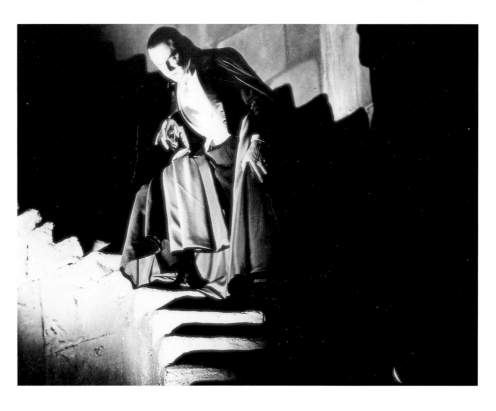

Turquoise and pink

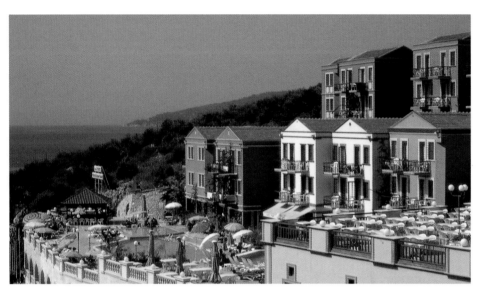

Turquoise is a blend of green and blue. It is so named because the Turks were fond of the colour and decorated many of their buildings with turquoise ceramic glazed tiles. Turquoise has the calming, expansive nature of green and the cool, quiet flow of blue. It can bring to mind a particular quality in the sky before or after sunset, a calm, warm sea, a beautiful lagoon, a pure mountain stream or distant hills in the mellow light of late summer.

functions of turquoise

The energy of turquoise allows the expression of our wishes. The green quality of growth is added to the blue quality of communication. Turquoise is the colour of the desire for freedom to be a unique individual. The blue ingredient ensures that, whatever the need may be in the heart of the individual, it will communicate itself and be recognized for what it is. Turquoise

△ **Turquoise and pink are both blends of colours that can be warm and cool. Both balance and strengthen life-energy at many levels.**

▽ **The Turks were skilled tilemakers and with access to the mines of Persia they were able to use turquoise pigments to great effect**.

USING TURQUOISE
Throughout the world turquoise stones have been used as protective amulets for promoting health and guarding against harm. A large proportion of everyone's energy comes from the turquoise motivation to experience life to the full. Wear turquoise jewellery to give yourself confidence and strength. Turquoise has a strengthening influence on all systems of the body bringing a sense of inner confidence.

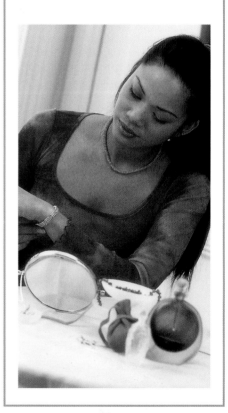

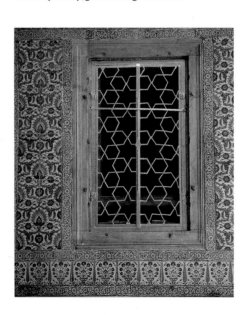

▽ **Turquoise is a copper ore with varying degrees of blue and green. Each mine produces a slight variation of colour.**

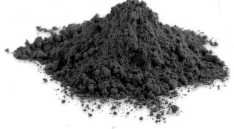

also represents the exploration of information through feelings and emotions. This creates the possibility for new interpretations of established ways for doing things, of new uses for old ideas.

Space and freedom are essential for every living creature. Restriction of natural behav-

iour patterns and the inability to find a place in the community cause a rapid build-up of stress and toxins in the body. This leads to a decrease in energy and greater susceptibility to disease. Turquoise can help when there is low energy, a lack of interest in life, a failure to fit in with the surroundings or a lack of courage to strike out on your own.

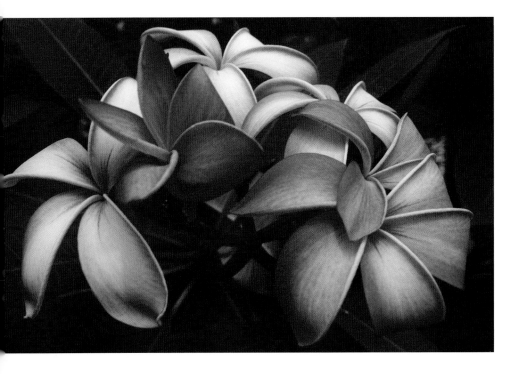

◁ Dark pink, bubble-gum pink and magenta are much more stimulating than pale tints. They provide the energy to make changes to improve one's life and are dynamic and assertive.

functions of pink

Pink is red and white combined in varying degrees. The quality of the energy will depend on how much red vibration is present. White is the potential for fullness, and red is the motivation to achieve that potential, so pink is a colour that promotes both these energies together.

Pink gives an underlying confidence to existence, it provides a level of support that means that it has the ability to neutralize any negative or destructive tendencies. Aggressive behaviour patterns arise where there is fear at an emotional level, or friction at a physical or mental level. Pink

▽ Pink promotes relaxation and acceptance of where one is in life without false views or feelings of complacency.

provides sufficient energy to move out of that negative state and enough clarity to recognize and clear away misconceptions.

Deep shades of pink that veer towards magenta have proved to be extremely effective in situations of disorder and violence, such as in prisons and police cells. In places such as these, a limited exposure to pink

light rapidly defuses aggressive attitudes and behaviour. These deeper shades of pink can also help to improve self-confidence and assertiveness, while pink's paler shades are more protective, promoting peace and being supportive of self-acceptance and feelings of self-worth.

Pink is sometimes seen only as a soft, feminine colour, a colour representing the qualities of caring and tenderness. It will also help to take the heat out of any turbulent or aggressive situation. The dynamic mix of red and white is a useful balance of male and female energies that can also be valuable as a healing colour, reducing the effects of disease as well as the fear and anguish disease can cause. Pink can help where other colours may have drawbacks, as it fundamentally supports the integrity of an individual.

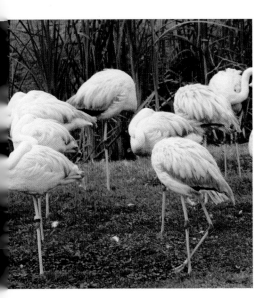

USING PINK

In any aggressive or threatening situation, or where there are simple misunderstandings leading to anger, visualizing pink around everyone can help to calm the mood and reduce tension.

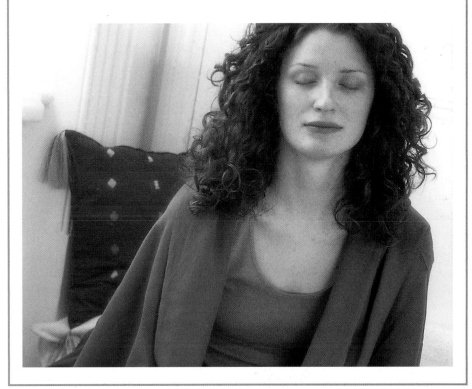

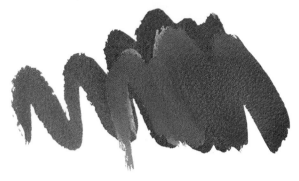

Brown and grey

Brown clothes were worn by the large majority of manual workers until the introduction of blue denim. As a mix of the primary colours, brown can blend into many surroundings. It is a disguise that shows no preference, no specific direction or attitude. It can be used very effectively to hide the true nature of the individual. Grey clothes are the favoured uniform of managers, businessmen and politicians. Grey reflects the desire to project coolness of mind, emotional stability and the ability to look down on the rest of the world with a detached neutrality. It epitomizes the myth of efficiency.

practical brown

Brown is a mixture of red, yellow and blue. Like every colour, brown has a wide range of shades and tones, each having a different effect. It is primarily a colour of the earth and the natural world. Brown acts as a solid background colour, a base upon which other, more striking colours can arise. As a combination, brown is neutral and non-threatening. Its warm tones are comfortable and familiar.

The red content makes brown a colour of practical energy and this mixed with the mental qualities of yellow and blue can encourage study and focus of the mind. However, in too great a quantity brown can also have a dulling effect, as it lacks the overall clarity to break out of established patterns of behaviour. Brown gives a state of solidity and reality from which one can grow. It suggests reliability and the desire to remain in the background, unnoticed.

In the traditional surroundings of an oak-panelled library or study, brown aids the transformation of inspiration and thoughts into practical, everyday reality. Discoveries and inventions need time devoted to painstaking detail, and involve going over the same set of ideas repeatedly until a solution emerges. Brown acts as a supporting colour in this process.

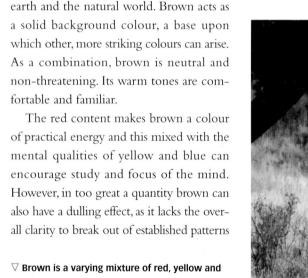

◁ **Brown is a warm, comfortable colour, reflecting wholesomeness, naturalness and dependability.**

▽ **Deer, like other forest or woodland animals, use their brown hides or coats to blend into the background and become virtually invisible.**

▽ **Brown is a varying mixture of red, yellow and blue. It can range from a burnt orange tone to a chocolate brown with hints of red and purple.**

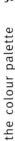

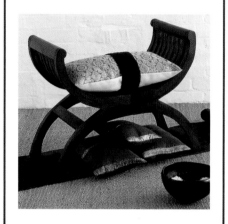
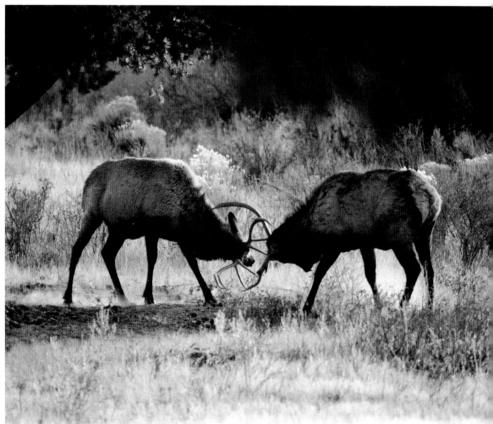

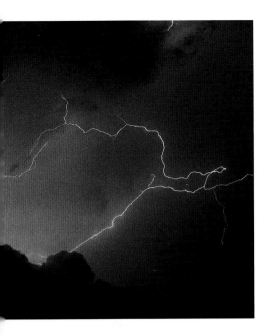

neutral grey

Grey is the true neutral colour. It is usually thought of as a combination of white and black, but a mixture of any complementary colours will produce grey. Grey is the colour of void, of emptiness, lack of movement, lack of emotion, lack of warmth, lack of any identifying characteristics in fact. Because of this, grey can be restful. If it contains a high proportion of white it will tend to take on the qualities of surrounding colours. If it has a greater amount of black, it can feel very heavy and depressing. Grey lacks information and this has a numbing effect on the mind, though not in a particularly peaceful way, as with blue or indigo. Indeed the inability to see into the colour can be reminiscent of the experience of fear or terror where decision-making processes seem frozen and even time stands still. With its emptiness, boredom and lack of direction, grey has an enervating and draining effect: its neutrality prevents us from moving towards an energetic state.

Unlike brown, grey has no connection to the solid earth or the life of nature.

▽ Grey pigments appear to be that colour because they scatter all light that hits them in a random way.

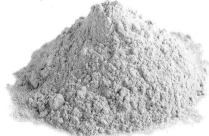

◁ Where grey skies are common they can have an oppressing influence on people as it reduces the intensity and effect of all other colours.

Immovable stone and cloudy skies reflect the impersonal, implacable nature of grey. Grey has a detached, isolated and unemotional feel. While brown suggests a down-to-earth practicality, grey has a cool, calculating mental neutrality, an unwillingness to get one's hands dirty.

Grey clothes can suggest that the wearer wishes to remain unsullied or uninvolved, but they can also suggest sophistication – being cool. When placed next to other colours, grey does have a cooling effect. It is moderating and stabilizing, making neighbouring colours stand out while muting their vibrational energy.

▽ Grey clothes suggest efficiency and are often used in the business world. Grey can also suggest a lack of imagination, however.

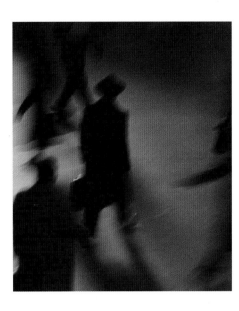

USING GREY

Grey clothing will emphasise neutrality. However, too much grey, or a wrong shade, will suggest lack of character, lack of initiative and extreme detachment. A hint of another colour that reflects individual preference will make all the difference: efficient, wellbehaved but with personality. If you want to emphasize your willingness to comply, wear grey.

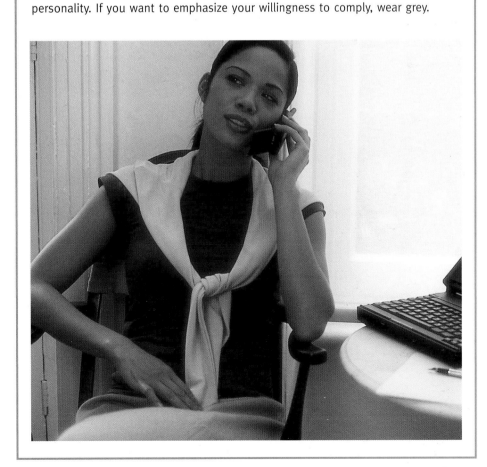

Self-healing
with Colour

An understanding of how the body uses the language of colour helps an individual to discover their personal colour needs. Selecting from a range of coloured, everyday items can provide unique guidance to enhance wellbeing, and provide guidance and clarity in life.

Human responses to colour

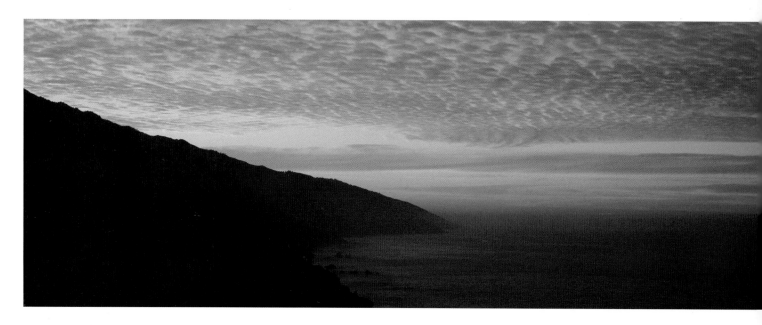

The only real difference between coloured light and any other radiation of the electromagnetic spectrum is that we can see it. Under the light of the sun, which reaches the earth with greatest strength in the visible spectrum, humankind has evolved to respond and make use of colour. The fact that the warm colours of reds and oranges activate and stimulate us while the cool colours of blues and violets calm us, probably derives from the biological triggers of daylight and nightfall.

eyes and light

Our eyes serve not only as a sense organ but also directly stimulate vitally important, fundamental and very primitive parts of the nervous system located deep in the brain. The hypothalamus, pituitary and pineal glands are all extremely light sensitive. Light reaching these areas of the brain has an immediate effect on the involuntary autonomic nervous system, changing our physical, mental and emotional states. The human eye is a complex and sophisticated

△ It is thought that our sensitivity to colour has evolved over time, in order to respond to the changing conditions of sunlight in our world.

sensing device. Light passes through the transparent lens and stimulates the retina at the back of the eyeball, which consists of specialized light-sensitive cells called rods and cones. The rods are sensitive to blue and green and work in dim light. The cones work best in daylight and are sensitive to different colours depending on the pigments

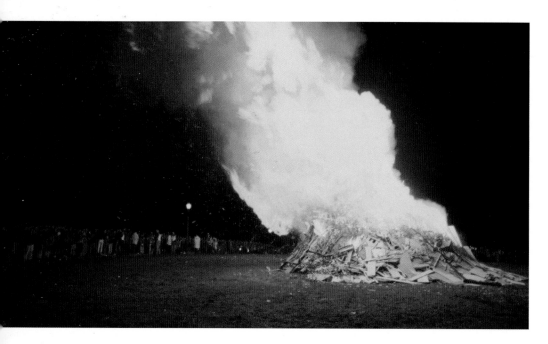

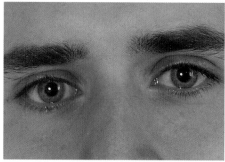

△ The human eye is one of the most complex structures in the whole animal kingdom, the product of millions of years of evolution.

◁ The warm colours in fire combine with the physical sense of heat, and promote feelings of warmth and comfort.

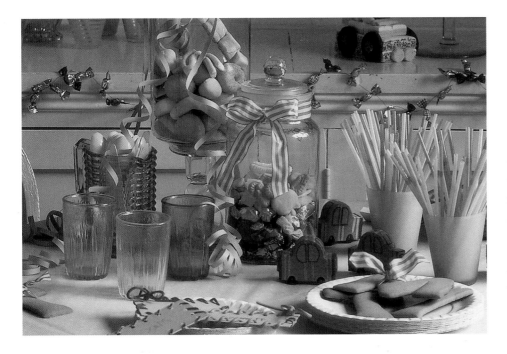

tors and healers can therefore find ways of using colour to manipulate our responses – for better or worse. Colour, as well as the amount of full-spectrum sunlight, has been shown to initiate profound changes in the nervous system. We are all moved by colour whether we are aware of the process or not, but increasing our knowledge of how colour influences us can help us to be aware of any attempts to manipulate us.

they contain. These photoelectric cells, when stimulated, send electrical impulses via the optic nerve into the brain where they are interpreted. The process of vision is primarily a function of the brain, for the eyes 'see' only a small area of the world at any one time. The eyeballs move very rapidly, 50 to 70 times a second, scanning the field of vision. It is the visual cortex in the brain that makes sense of this information and tells us what we are seeing.

△ Colour is the food of our emotions. It reflects our thoughts and moods consciously and unconsciously. Combinations of bright, festive colours, for example, are powerfully attractive, particularly to young children.

▽ Although we think of colour as a decorative, superficial thing, our choices and reactions are dictated by the energy each wavelength exerts on important areas of the unconscious brain.

NATURAL LIGHT

It has been recommended that people spend at least 20 minutes outside in direct sunlight every day. If you wear glasses or contact lenses it is also a good idea to remove them for five or ten minutes every few hours, in order to get the benefit of natural light.

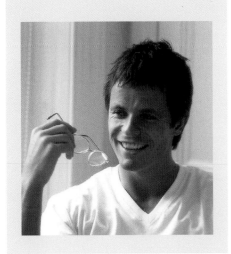

the energy of light

Light impulses do not go just to the visual cortex in the brain. Some nerves go from the retina directly to the hypothalamus, a small organ that regulates most of the life-sustaining functions of the body, such as control of the autonomic nervous system, energy levels, internal temperature, cycles of rest and activity, growth, circulation, breathing, reproduction and the emotions. The hypothalamus directly affects the pituitary gland, which is the major controlling organ for the endocrine system and all its hormonal secretions. Light from the eyes also directly affects the pineal gland, which modifies our behaviour patterns according to the amount of light it receives. The pineal gland regulates our energy so that we can remain in balance with our environment. The correspondences between the endocrine glands and the subtle energy systems of the body, indicate that colour affects all levels of our being.

The eyes are thus not simply a source of information about the world around us, they also allow light energy to be carried to the centre of the brain where it can create profound changes at the level of cellular function, physical activity, emotional and mental states. Advertisers, interior decora-

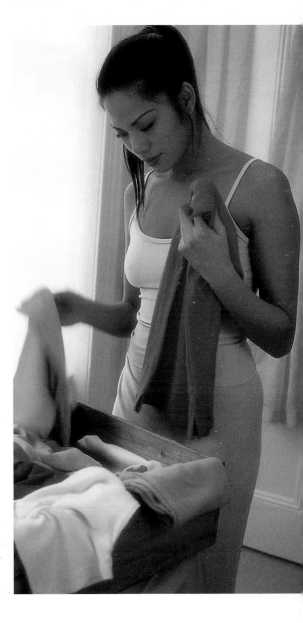

Light as healer

The sun is the motor that drives this world. A change to the energy we receive on the surface of the earth is like a change in gear that speeds up or slows down all life processes. It is not a matter of choice – life has evolved to take advantage of the energy of the sun and so is automatically connected to its cycles.

cycles of light

At sunrise, the sun low on the horizon is red. As it climbs into the sky, the widening angle with our point on the earth's surface allows more orange and then yellow light to reach the ground. Experimentation has clearly shown that red light increases blood pressure, pulse rate and breathing rate, and that these functions are further increased in orange light, reaching their peak in yellow light. The human physiological response to light has evolved so that the rising sun stimulates us into activity and alertness.

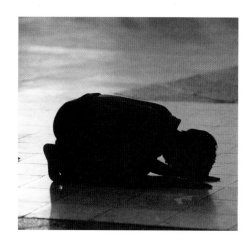

△ Sun, moon and stars are the earliest deities in many religions. Light is a universal metaphor for enlightenment and spiritual fulfilment.

Other experiments have shown a decrease in blood pressure, pulse rate and breathing rate when people are exposed to green light. Relaxation increases with blue light and is at its fullest in complete darkness. White light has been found to have similar quietening effects to blue light. As daylight fades the subduing green light changes to the blue of evening, then the

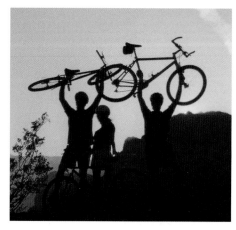

△ Energy levels, hormone activity and mood are all automatically regulated according to the quality of light.

darkness of night, with perhaps only the moon for illumination. Night is the natural time of rest and reflection. Emotionally and physiologically we respond to colours as they fit the times of the day, just as our distant forebears did before artificial light sources were available.

light reaction in cells

Studies with plants grown under different colours and ranges of light have demonstrated that the wrong kind of light can seriously damage their growth and health. Full-spectrum natural sunlight with normal levels of ultraviolet light (which is filtered out by most types of glass) is essential to maintain the normal, healthy functioning of plant cells. The same has been found with animal cells. Filtering light or exposure to a single colour for long periods causes cells to function abnormally and even eventually die. These studies seem to suggest that humans, as well as plants, need a balanced environment of light and colour. Until 1879 when the electric light bulb was invented, most people lived and worked outdoors in natural light. Now more and more people spend a large proportion of their lives in enclosed environments exposed to artificial light and completely cut off from the sun.

▽ Only the comparatively recent introduction of artificial lighting has changed our patterns of rest and activity, triggered by sunrise and sunset.

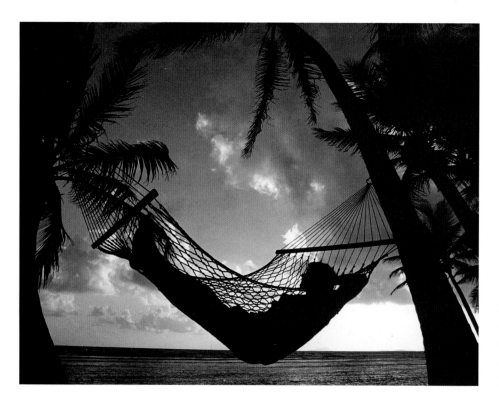

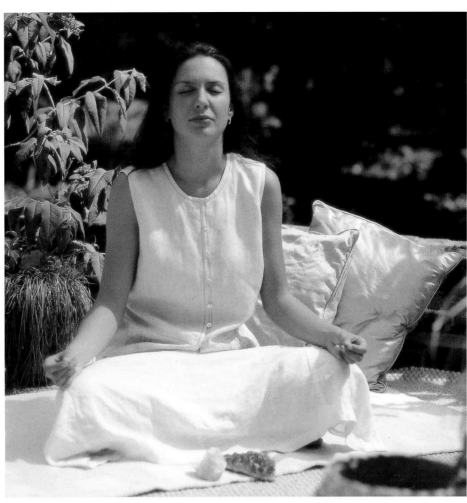

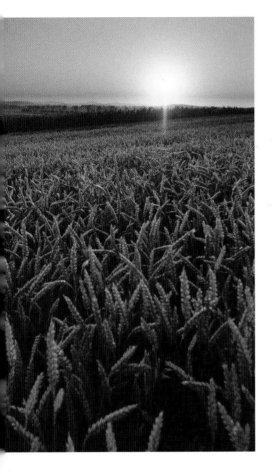

△ All life has evolved to take advantage of the different qualities of sunlight through the year.

trum light that resembles sunlight and which resets the chemical balance within the pineal gland, the organ that is disrupted. Without sufficient exposure to the full spectrum of light from the sun, the finely balanced chemical reactions in our bodies tend to falter, leaving us prone to ill health.

△ An indoor lifestyle may be a factor in our lack of health and sense of well-being. Spending time outside will counteract this.

▽ During the long winter months the grey rainy weather in some countries can contribute to feelings of seasonal depression.

When full-spectrum, balanced fluorescent lighting was tested in schools against normal white tubes, there appeared to be a significant decrease in irritability, hyperactivity and fatigue in students after just one month. Interestingly, there also seemed to be a correlation between poor quality lighting and the amount of tooth decay!

The reduction of sunlight on a cloudy day or, more profoundly, in the long months of winter, significantly changes the mood of most people, but for some, the lack of sunlight can be seriously debilitating. Seasonal Affective Disorder (or SAD) causes mood swings, low energy levels and depression that begins as the days grow shorter and only gradually improves with the onset of spring. Effective treatment is by exposure each day to several hours of bright full-spec-

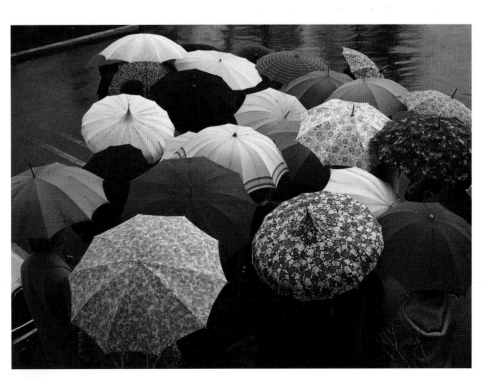

Single colour guidance

Our instinctive emotional response to colour can tell us a lot about ourselves. It reflects back to us how we are functioning. It can show life-long tendencies, immediate situations or a potential direction in personal development. Sometimes certain colours stay with us as favourites for many years. This is reflected in the colours we choose to paint our home, inside and out, and the predominant colours in our wardrobe. It is possible to interpret these colour preferences through their known correspondences to our physical, emotional, mental and even spiritual state.

colour choice

Given a range of colours to choose from, the process of self-reflection and self-revelation can begin. The simplest approach is to make spontaneous choices:

1. Which colour do you like the most?
2. Which colour do you like the least?

The colour you like the most will, as likely as not, be present in your home or in

▽ **Sometimes our instinctive choice of food reflects our energy needs of the moment.**

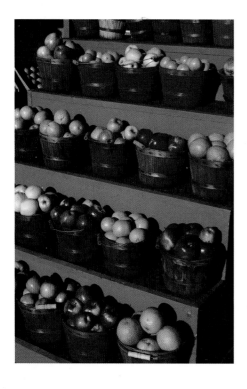

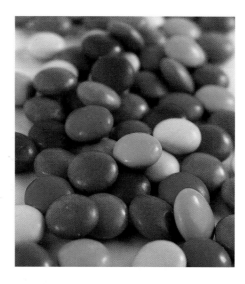

△ **Coloured sweets can be used as a way of identifying colour energies that are lacking.**

▷ **Flowers, with their vibrant colour and variety of shape, are an excellent way to introduce a balancing colour into the surroundings.**

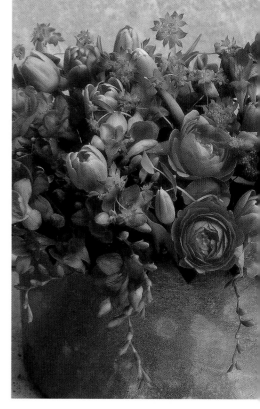

your clothes. It may also be a colour that you need to help you in a current situation. By looking at the full range of correspondences for that colour, as discussed earlier in this book, you may get insight into a new direction in life. However, if the colour you have chosen is an absolute favourite and you have no desire to reflect on other choices, you may have become stuck in particular habit patterns. Again, look at the correspondences for that colour to see what these habits might be.

The colour you like least will suggest areas of your life that may require attention and healing. Each colour has positive as well as negative attributes, so it is a good idea to bring the positive energy of a colour you dislike into your life to create balance. Do this through new activities, the choice of food, by wearing that colour in clothing or adding it to your surroundings.

The process of self-analysis through colour can be developed a step further by deciding, before you make your choices, what each choice will represent. For exam-

ple, a series of three choices could be selected to show:

1. What your physical needs are now (e.g. activities, food, clothes)
2. What your emotional needs are now (e.g. peace, space, fun, company)
3. What your mental needs are now (e.g. time to study, standing up for yourself)

how to do it

1. Collect together a selection of different coloured items, for example ribbon lengths, pieces of card or buttons so that you have at least one of each colour of the rainbow plus a selection of other colours.
2. Lay the items out at random on a plain background.
3. Close your eyes and have in your mind your first question.
4. Relax, open your eyes and pick up the colour that you are immediately, and instinctively drawn to.
5. Repeat these steps for each of your questions in turn.

what does it mean?

The colour that you have instinctively selected will give you the answer in the language of colour. You can then introduce the colour energy into your life by whichever means seem appropriate. The colour choices may highlight some aspects of your life that have not been clear to you. This process can bring issues to the surface so they can be looked at and healed.

taking it further

You can invent any number of permutations for a series of questions or choices. For example:

1. Where am I now?
2. What are my main difficulties?
3. What is at the root of those difficulties?
4. What are my priority needs?
5. What is the next possible step and the way forward?

The colour choices can be interpreted through colour correspondences and then introduced into your life using the information in this book.

▽ Use collections of differently coloured items, such as ribbons or pieces of fabric, for single colour guidance exercises.

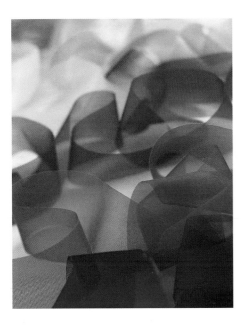

CHOOSING COLOURS

Try not to think about the choice you make. Just pay attention to where your eyes settle as soon as they are open. For a moment or two you may find your eyes just scan over the colours, but soon they will focus on one in particular.

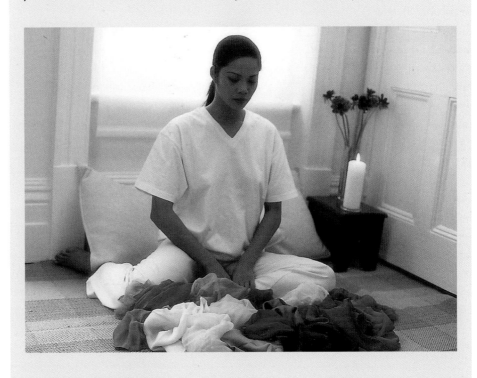

△ Lay out all your colours so that your eyes can easily scan all of them at the same time.

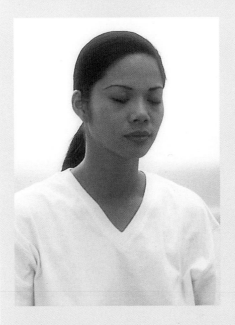

△ Close your eyes, take a moment to relax, and think of the area you wish to investigate.

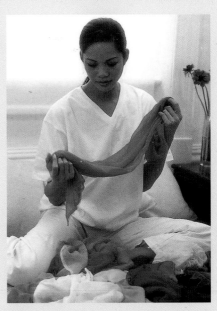

△ When you feel ready, open your eyes and pick the colour that first draws your attention.

single colour assessment

A simple way to determine your day-to-day colour needs is to carry out a single colour assessment. This process can be done as often as you like. Sit quietly with these pages open in front of you and go through the steps below one by one.

how to assess yourself

1. Cover the chart showing the keys to colours with a sheet of paper. This helps to stop the logical and judgmental part of the mind from interfering with the instinctive choice of colour.

2. Note down on a piece of paper the number of choices you will make and what each will represent. For example, a one-colour choice could represent what you most need today; a two-colour choice could reveal firstly a problem you are encountering, and secondly, a possible solution.

3. With the framework decided, close your eyes. For each choice, open your eyes and record the colour that your eyes are immediately drawn to.

▽ **Relax before starting a single colour assessment and remember that you are being guided towards a colour by your intuition.**

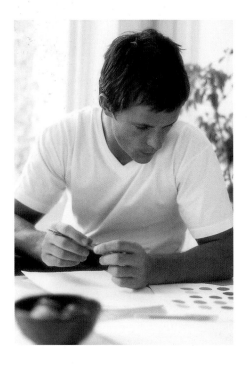

4. Repeat the process for each choice, then look up the correspondences on the chart.

5. Consider the questions and phrases linked to each of your colour choices, and where appropriate, decide to bring that colour more into your life.

▷ **Any coloured items can be used for colour assessment. The important thing is to decide on an appropriate framework of questions.**

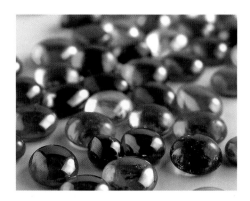

KEYS TO COLOURS	
Colour	**Key phrases and questions that may help you to focus ideas**
Dark red	Need to keep your feet on the ground What is taking your attention away from where it needs to be?
Red	Need to take action, now What is stopping you doing what is necessary?
Orange	Need to let go of old, worn out ideas, things, emotions What is blocking you? What are you allowing to block your way?
Gold	Need to relax, enjoy life What is making you doubt yourself?
Yellow	Need to start thinking clearly What are you afraid of?
Olive green	Need to reassess where you are going What hidden factors are stopping your growth?
Green	Need for space to gain fresh perspective What is restricting you?
Turquoise	Need to put into words exactly what you feel What are your strengths?
Light blue	Need to talk to people around you What do you need to express to others?
Dark blue	Need for peace and time on your own What are you so close to that you cannot see clearly what is happening?
Violet	Need to heal yourself What are you sacrificing to appear as a 'good' or 'helpful' person?
Black	Need to be quiet and listen What are you wanting to hide from?
White	Need to make some changes What is painful to look at in the real world?
Pink	Need to look after yourself more What thoughts do you have about yourself that are too critical?
Magenta	Need to take time out to repair all levels of yourself What have you been overdoing at the expense of your own health?
Brown	Need to focus on the practicalities of life In what areas of your life have you been too dreamy?
Grey	Need to disappear into the background What do you want to hide and why?

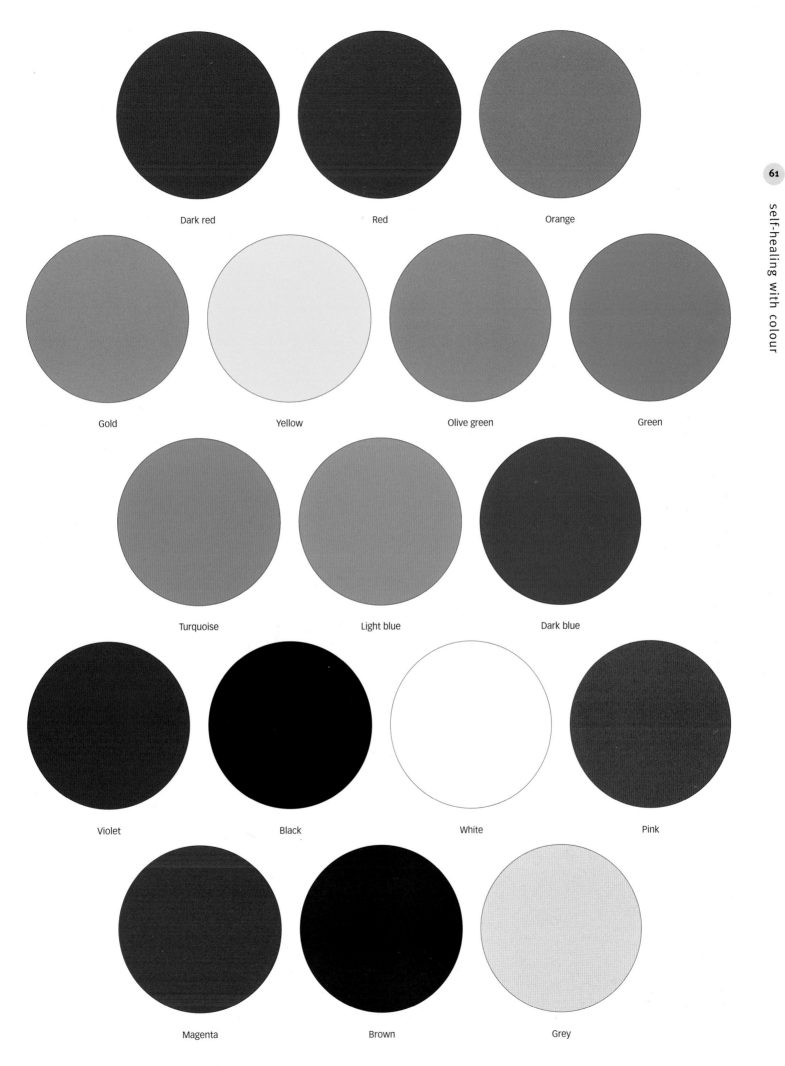

Dark red

Red

Orange

Gold

Yellow

Olive green

Green

Turquoise

Light blue

Dark blue

Violet

Black

White

Pink

Magenta

Brown

Grey

Specific colour placement

In certain situations it is helpful to introduce specific colours into the environment for immediate short-term effect. This can often be more effective than redecorating whole rooms, or enthusiastically pursuing certain foods or activities. Once the situation changes, the colour can be removed until it is needed again in the future.

everyday uses of colour

When you use visualization techniques for relaxation and stress removal, it can sometimes be difficult to return to everyday activities or focus on practical tasks, especially if your experience has been deep. The same problem sometimes occurs in people who meditate regularly, as returning to the realities of the world can be disruptive. A rich red object such as a cushion or a piece of fabric can help. After relaxation or meditation, try gazing at the colour red for about a minute. This will integrate the benefits of meditation into your body and prepare you to return to the normal world.

Students studying for examinations will find the process less tiring and generally more effective if they introduce a shade of yellow into their study-space. An acid yellow will keep the mind alert, while sunshine yellow combines alertness with relaxation.

▽ **Small areas of bright colour, like cushion covers, are excellent ways to temporarily bring colour energy into a room.**

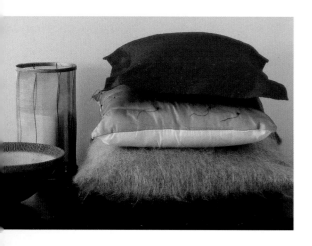

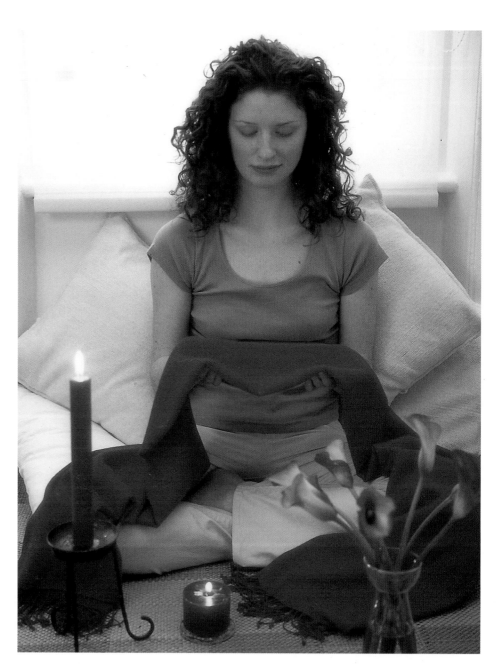

colour and reading difficulties

American psychologist Helen Irlen introduced the idea of reading through coloured overlays in 1988. Her attention was drawn to a type of dyslexia called SSS or Scotopic Sensitivity Syndrome. People with this difficulty are very light-sensitive. They have trouble dealing with high contrasts, such as black and white, find that letters and numbers 'move' on the page and have difficulty with groups of letters or numbers. They also

△ **Having a red object in a meditation space helps to ground spiritual energies at a practical level. Tibetan monks often wear red shawls or robes for this purpose.**

have a poor attention span. Irlen has devised a series of tests for people with reading difficulties which enables her to help them by recommending reading through different coloured overlays or tinted spectacle lenses. These measures can alleviate, or even sometimes remove the problem entirely. Irlen's

THE WORK OF BARBARA MEISTER VITALE

Barbara Meister Vitale, a well-known educator and lecturer in the USA, has used colour in her work since 1970. During her research with children and the way they learn, she has concluded that:

• Lots of different coloured pieces of material in the classroom help to reduce hyperactivity and increase children's attention span.

• Children behave differently when dressed in different coloured clothes.

• Using several different coloured pens and coloured paper increases children's learning skills and aids their ability to recall.

• Using a blue light helps both adults and children in their reading and studying.

• People with reading difficulties respond well when a transparent colour overlay is placed on their reading material.

• The effect of colour is unique to each individual. It might be their favourite colour, or its complementary colour, that is most helpful to them.

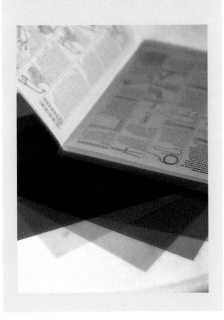

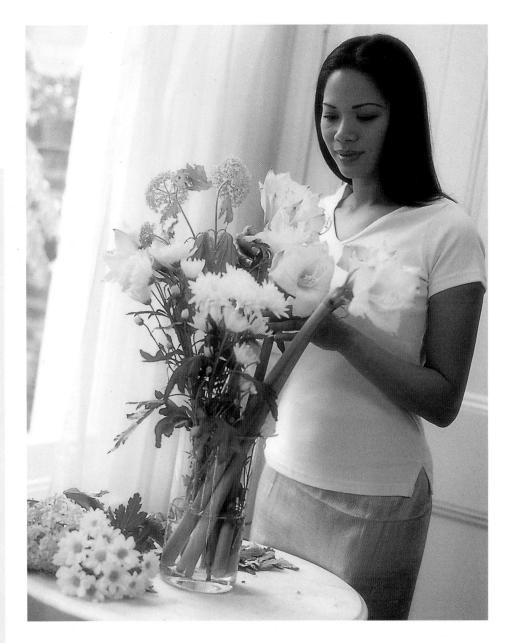

△ **Bringing colour into a space is more than a design or fashion whim. Colour has an impact on every activity around it.**

▽ **Study can be helped by having objects of lemon yellow around that help the memory functions of the brain. If exam-stress is a problem, a bright golden yellow encourages relaxation and reduces nervousness.**

work has centred on people with SSS, who make up approximately one-fifth of those with dyslexia or other identified learning difficulties. Irlen believes, however, that her findings could benefit a much wider section of people, and that about one-fifth of the general population could benefit from reading through colour. There is medical evidence to suggest that wearing coloured lenses can also reduce the incidence of migraine by up to 80%.

The benefits of using colour in health and in education are only now being investigated scientifically. Perhaps in the future these inexpensive and simple tools could help in many situations, and may well transform many peoples lives.

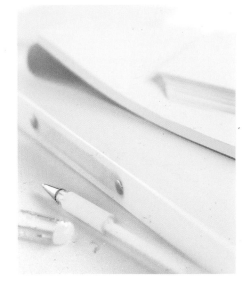

Colour in Foods

Bringing colour into our lives through the food
we eat is one of the most powerful uses of colour
as a healing tool. Each colour represents coded
information, giving guidance to the nutritional
content of a food. The colour code can also
indicate the effect of that food on the body.

Rainbow diet

Each of us has colours that we prefer and some that we dislike. Any reaction of an emotional nature to colour, either positive or negative, can indicate how colour can be used to promote healing and wellbeing.

A balance of attractive colours in the food we eat plays a large part in a healthy diet. But few people recognize their instinctive reaction to the colour of food, or notice that they get drawn towards that colour in a foodstore or marketplace. Manufacturers of convenience foods play on this reaction, which is why many packaged foods contain dyes and colourings to tempt our palate.

The effect of a food is not always gauged by the colour we see; its colour-related action or quality is also important. One of the qualities of orange is to eliminate toxins. Brown rice and oats are good detoxifiers, so can be described as having an

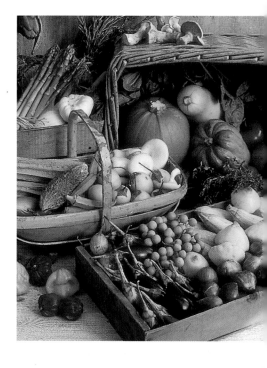

△ **Fresh fruit and vegetables provide a banquet of colours to feast the eyes and tempt the poorest of appetites.**

orange action. Often the body tries to direct us to the foods we need to rebalance our health. It is worth observing the types of food that appeal to someone after an illness or shock. Allowed a free choice we will always tend to be drawn to the foods we need by colour as much as by smell or taste but we rarely recognise or allow ourselves to follow through and eat the foods.

▽ **Unprocessed natural sugars could be thought of as better for us than the white, processed varieties. We do, however, get enough sugar for our daily needs from eating fruits and vegetables without having to add it to other foods.**

CHOOSING FOOD BY COLOUR

• Foods that display our favourite colours will always be needed because they give us the particular energy that supports our body's function.

• Foods belonging to the least-favourite, or even hated, colours will provide the nutrition and colour energy that we are lacking.

• Food colours that we are attracted to temporarily reflect the immediate nutritional needs of the body.

• If you have problems that correspond to certain colours, you may wish to introduce foods of that colour into your diet to help your body with its healing.

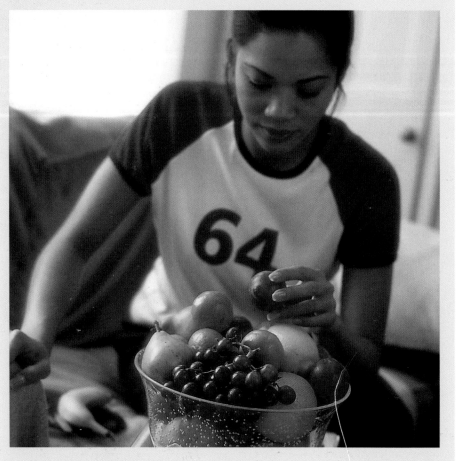

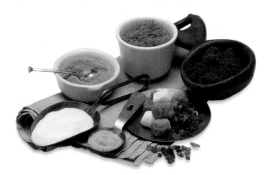

RED FOODS AND FOODS THAT WORK IN A RED WAY

Red foods are generally rich in minerals and provide good sources of protein. They are good for increasing levels of vitality. Red deficiencies are shown through low energy levels, anaemia, light-headedness and lack of stamina.

Foods have different kinds of colour energy, one is its obvious outwards appearance, the colour it actually is, another is the inherent energy it supplies. Chocolate is a good example of this, although not red in colour it is an important red energy food because of the instant energy it supplies. In appearance watercress and parsley are both green foods, but their high levels of minerals give them a red quality. Red wine is red in colour and provides iron, but its high alcohol level means that it also provides violet energy, so it can be classed in either colour category.

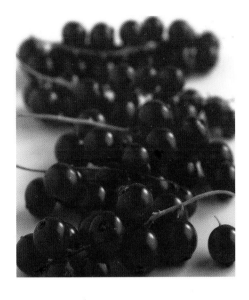

△ **Redcurrants are widely used to accompany rich, red foods, such as meat and game.**

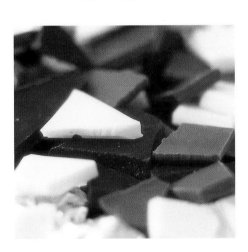

△ **Chocolate is an important red energy food as it gives instant energy.**

Red fruits	Strawberries, raspberries, cherries
Red vegetables	Red cabbage, beetroot, radishes, peppers, onions, tomatoes, chillies, watercress, parsley
Other red foods	Meat, pulses, nuts, fish
red vitamins	B12 (vital for the absorption of iron)
red minerals	Iron (helps the blood to carry oxygen), magnesium (good for nerve responses, cell energy, hormones, healthy bones), zinc (good for fertility; healthy hair, skin and nails)
Other red nutrients	Fatty acids (improve function of cells and promote healthy blood, skin, hair and nails)
Red non-foods (foods with little or no nutritional value)	Red wine (stimulates and relaxes in moderation), coffee (stimulates the adrenals, diuretic), chocolate (gives instant energy), sugar, the ultimate non-food (very addictive but gives instant short-lived energy, followed by a big energy 'low')

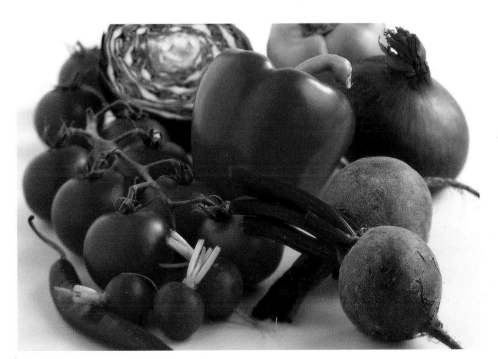

◁ **Red foods can be very attractive when energies are low or following periods of illness.**

▽ **Soft red fruit is many people's favourite way of absorbing red energy and natural sugars.**

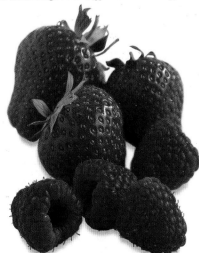

ORANGE FOODS AND FOODS THAT WORK IN AN ORANGE WAY

Orange foods help with the release of toxins and stress from the body, they support the reproductive system and encourage creativity at all levels. Orange deficiencies are shown in constipation, artist's block, difficulties with fertility and stiffness of the joints. Orange foods help with the release

Orange fruits	Oranges, peaches, apricots
Orange vegetables	Pumpkin, peppers, carrots
Other orange foods	Brown rice, sesame seeds, oats (provides roughage which is mucilaginous and gentle), shellfish
orange vitamins	Vitamin A (for healthy eyes, skin, stable energy levels), vitamin C (strengthens cells and blood vessels, helps absorption of iron)
orange minerals	Calcium (for muscle relaxation and healthy bones), copper (helps absorption of iron, improves flexibility of arteries), selenium (free-radical scavenger, helps reduce the effects of ageing), zinc (for healthy reproductive organs)

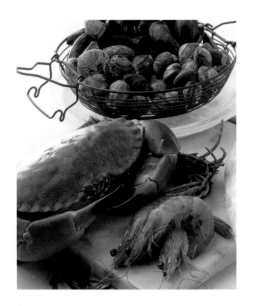

◁ Seafood is rich in many trace minerals and Omega 3 fatty acids that support the reproductive system.

▷ Oranges contain the key nutrient Vitamin C and carotenoids that support the body in healing the effects of disease and ageing.

foods into a system that is tired or toxic is easier for the body to handle than the strong, direct energy of red foods that could appear on first glance to be the solution.

▽ The vitamin C and zinc in carrots provide an excellent combination to help the body detoxify metals and other pollutants.

of toxins and stress from the body by encouraging the system to become more efficient in the natural elimination and excretory processes. This, in turn, aids relaxation and the release of stress as the body lets go of unwanted and waste products.

Orange foods contain key nutrients that support and maintain the reproductive systems. These foods can also aid the flow of creativity on other levels too.

Lack of orange and orange-energy foods can be evident in physical constipation, but also in stagnation in other areas, such as artist's block and stiffness in muscles and joints. Introducing orange or orange-energy

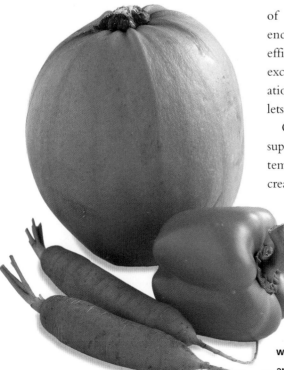

◁ We are often attracted to orange foods when our bodies need to release significant amounts of stress or toxicity.

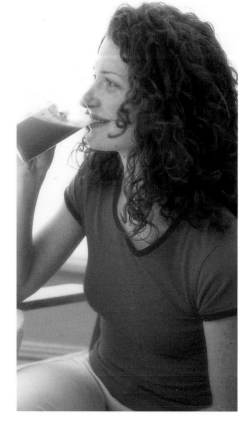

YELLOW FOODS AND FOODS THAT WORK IN A YELLOW WAY

The sun gives us our main source of yellow during daylight hours, but as modern life uses up the yellow vibration in dealing with pollution, chemicals, living indoors and high stress levels, yellow foods are needed in large amounts by much of the industrialized world's population.

Lack of yellow leads to irritability, tension, poor memory, restlessness, inefficient absorption of nutrients, digestive problems,

▷ Bananas are rich in potassium that helps to maintain healthy muscles. Grapefruit and lemons help to fight infections.

▽ Yellow foods are a useful addition to the diet for those who are studying, or coping with worries that they can do little about.

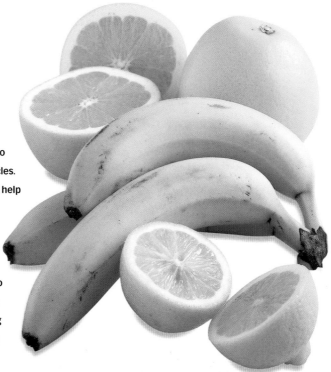

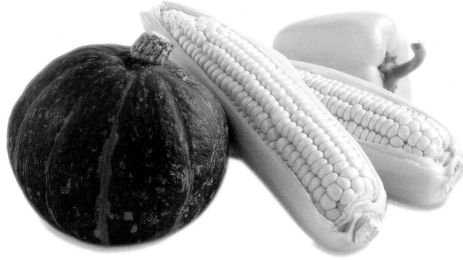

a drop in immunity, a tendency towards hot flushes, feelings of depression, and inability to make decisions.

Problems with learning, concentration and memory can indicate a lack of yellow energy in the body. Sometimes this lack is made worse by the modern lifestyle, lighting and high levels of stress. However, recent research into learning and attention difficulties has concluded that fish oils (Omega 3 fatty acids) have a crucial role in the internal body chemistry. The systems of people experiencing these problems seem to be unable to assimilate these vital nutrients correctly. This indicates that what were once thought of as behavioural problems are actually difficulties with nutrition. Giving children experiencing these problems daily supplements of fatty acids – a yellow food – resulted in significant improvement in over 40% of cases, confirming the research.

▽ Grains that are made into flours form the staple diets of most cultures.

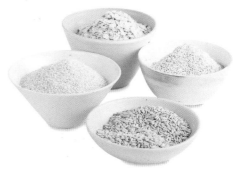

Yellow fruits	Lemon, bananas, grapefruit
Yellow vegetables	Grains (rice, corn, wheat, rye etc.), peppers, pumpkins
Other foods	Eggs, fish, oils, food rich in fatty acids
Vitamins	Vitamin A (for healthy tissues, blood, eyes and immune system), vitamin B complex (helps the body to convert food into energy, support nerves and muscles), vitamin D (for absorption of calcium, promotes healthy muscles, nerves and parathyroid), vitamin E (antioxidant, good for healthy tissues and wound repair)
Minerals	Sodium and potassium (for healthy blood pressure, cell function, smooth muscle function), selenium (for smooth skin, protects blood cells), phosphorus (for healthy bones, teeth, kidneys, nerves and energy levels), iodine (for balanced function of thyroid, healthy arteries), chromium (helps metabolism of sugars and the function of the pancreas), molybdenum (facilitates use of iron and fats), manganese (stabilizes hormones, improves nerve function)
Non-foods	Food additives (interfere with natural digestive processes), alcohol (depletes the liver of nutrients, overworks the pancreas), sugar (overworks the pancreas)

▷ One serving a day of green leafy, raw vegetables is thought to be the minimum for a healthy body.

GREEN FOODS AND FOODS THAT WORK IN A GREEN WAY

Food that is green, or that works in a green way, tends to be rich in vitamins and minerals, though these can be lost in cooking or storage. Some parts of the world do not support the growing of fresh green foods, so people living in these places have to find

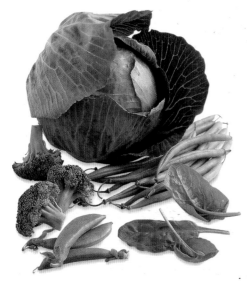

△ Dark, leafy greens are some of the best sources of vitamins and anti-oxidants, that help us to deal with old or dysfunctional cells throughout the body.

▽ Green foods calm our emotions, by providing the nutrients that the body uses to balance all of our energies.

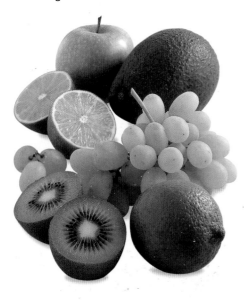

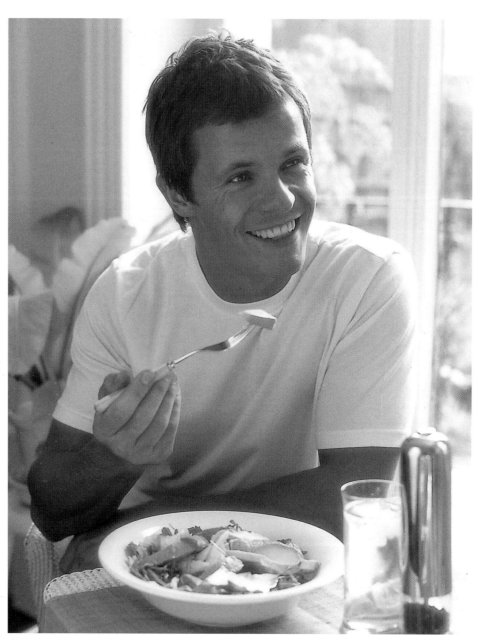

other sources of green nutrients. The Inuit people of northern Canada, for example, live on a diet almost entirely based on fish and fish products, which supply the green energy they need. All minerals act in a green way and all therapeutic herbs, as well as culinary ones, also come under this heading.

Lack of a green vibration creates depression, a feeling of being trapped, breathing difficulties and a lack of self-value. Being in a large space, in the open air, and among natural surroundings is a quick way to bring a green vibration into your life if you feel your green food intake is insufficient.

Eating foods in their natural season, or where possible, foods grown locally, allow the body to settle into the rhythms and patterns of our immediate surroundings.

Many leafy green foods are categorised as bitters by nutritionalists as they stimulate the liver and help to keep the whole of the digestive system in balance.

Green fruits	Apples, pears, avocados, green grapes, limes, kiwifruit
Green vegetables	Cabbage, calabrese, broccoli, kale, sprouts, green beans, peas, leeks, spinach
Other foods	Most culinary herbs – marjoram, basil, oregano
Vitamins/minerals	All vitamins and minerals

Blue and violet fruits	Plums, blueberries, black grapes
Blue energy vegetables	Kelp and all seaweed products, asparagus
Violet vegetables	Purple sprouting broccoli, aubergines
Violet energy herbs	St John's wort (acts on the pineal gland)
Blue and violet energy vitamins	Vitamin E (stabilizes oxygen in the body, improves pituitary gland function)
Blue energy minerals	Iodine (enhances the function of the thyroid gland)
Violet energy minerals	Potassium (stabilizes electrolytes in the body, keeps oxygen supplied to the brain)

BLUE AND VIOLET FOODS AND FOODS THAT WORK IN A BLUE AND VIOLET WAY

There are very few foods that are blue or violet coloured. However, some foods work in a blue or violet way. Blue foods are useful when the voice, glands and organs of the neck, and communication skills need help. Violet vibration foods have a remarkable effect on the workings of the mind.

negative violet effects

Food additives and colourings serve to create illusion (a violet function) and relate to the shelf-life or appearance of foods. Some

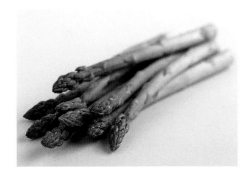

△ **Good crops of asparagus need special fertilizers, usually seaweed or from a seaweed source, to ensure an adequate supply of iodine.**

▽ **Dark-coloured grapes produce varying shades of red wine. The violet qualities of otherworldliness are encountered when drinking too much.**

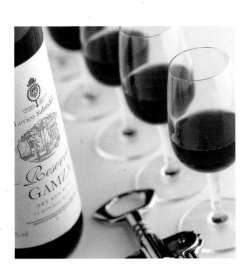

▷ **Purple and violet foods bring unusual colouring to dishes or culinary displays.**

additives also have an addictive quality, a trait that also belongs to a violet vibration. Both alcohol and sugar belong in this violet category when they are used in excess to escape from the reality of the world. Alcohol in particular is often the socially acceptable face of addiction and escapism.

Genetically modified foods also reflect a violet vibration because of the false idealism associated with their production. They are being upheld as the solution to world hunger, when in reality, there is already more than enough food to go around, but it is not being shared and distributed appropriately.

healers and intoxicants

Plants that have a violet resonance have long been used in healing all over the world. When used carefully under experienced supervision they can open the consciousness to other realms of experience. The use of intoxicants is a topic where cultures clash and legal entanglements abound, creating confusion and subversion which are strong violet traits.

In Meso-American traditions, a small cactus plant called peyote (*Lophophora williamsii*) is ritually harvested and widely used for its mind-expanding effects in religious and healing ceremonies.

Throughout the region of the Amazon basin a vine grows called ayahuasca (*Banesteriopsis caapi*) that is collected from the forest, cut into small sections and boiled for many hours with combinations of other plants. Ayahuasca too, is an intoxicant used in healing and religious ceremonies, though it requires a special preliminary diet to give maximum benefit. Both ayahuasca and peyote are valued as purifiers of the body and are used to remove the causes of infection and illness.

Basil, the common pot-herb, used in Mediterranean cooking, has specific and therapeutic effects when taken in small amounts. Drunk as a tea, it can help relax the body while keeping the mind alert.

▽ **Purple basil belongs to the same family as holy basil, which is used in the Indian subcontinent as a sacred herb of meditation.**

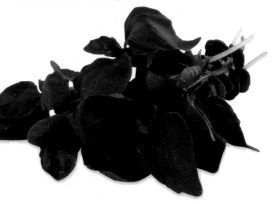

Colour Therapies

Colour has been used as a therapeutic tool for thousands of years. Today many of the traditional uses of colour for healing have changed little. The original practices have created a firm foundation for new ideas and applications of colour in the quest for health and wellbeing.

Theories of colour healing

Colour has always been associated with certain types of energy that are useful to both the healer and the magician. In the Middle Ages, colour was one of the correspondences used in magic along with planets, elements, spirits and angelic beings, metals, herbs, shapes and numbers. Tibetan and Chinese traditional medicine requires knowledge of the relationship between the colours of the elements and the compass directions to balance health. Yet it was only in the 19th century that science began to verify the healing possibilities of colour.

The German natural philosopher J.W. von Goethe (1749–1832) greatly influenced 19th-century ideas about light and colour. His book *Die Farben Lehre* (*The Theory of Colour*), published in 1810, combined scientific observation with metaphysical concepts, describing colour as an interplay

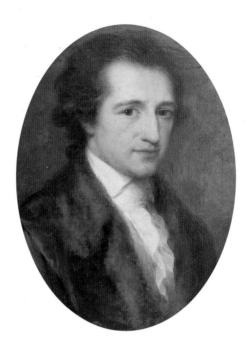

△ As an artist and scientist, Goethe was an important influence on colour theory.

of the polarities of light and dark. Goethe saw colour as an expression of spirituality and a way of expressing the inner nature of humanity. His thinking influenced artists such as Turner and teachers like Rudolph Steiner, who became influential in forming the colour theories of the 20th century.

During the 19th century there was an increasing interest in the healing properties of light. In 1851 Jacob Lorber wrote *The Healing Power of Sunlight*, which advocated exposing diseased parts of the body to the sun's rays as well as taking sun-charged mineral water and even sun-energized salt and other substances for speedier healing. In 1877 the American physician Dr Seth

▽ As in the 19th century, sunlight is still seen as part of the healing process today, and is often used as a therapeutic tool.

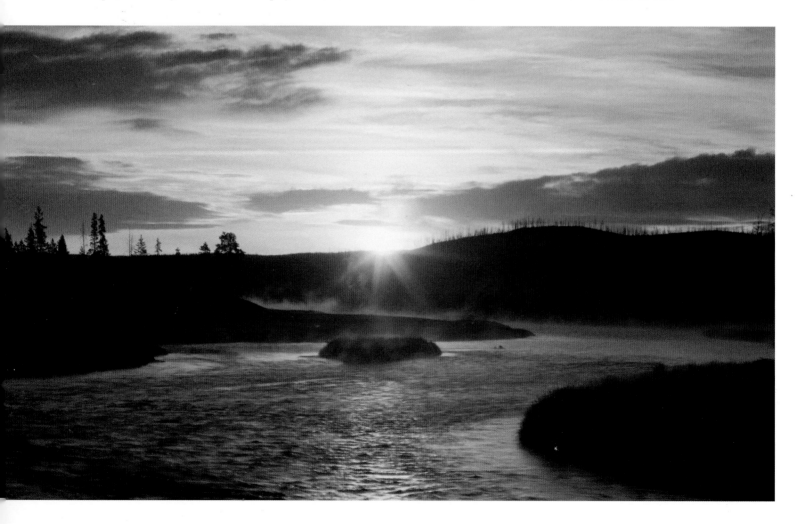

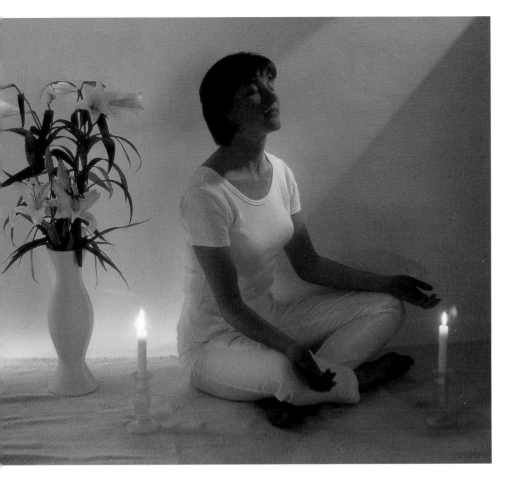

◁ **Blue light has been found to significantly reduce the pain of a form of arthritis – the longer the exposure the better the results.**

▽ **Gradual and consistent exposure to yellow light decreases blood pressure and heart rate and increases energy and endurance.**

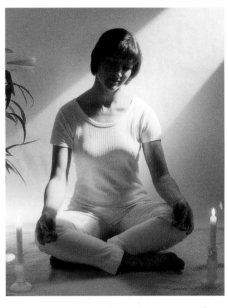

Pancoast published *Blue and Red Lights*, in which he discussed using coloured filters to alter the body's function. He found that red filtered light would energize the nervous system while blue would sedate it. A year later, in *The Principles of Light and Colour*, another American physician, Dr Edwin Babitt, focused on the healing properties of the three primary colours. He began by creating small cabinets through which he shone filtered sunlight on to his patients. He later developed ways of projecting electric light through filters on to the patient. Babitt also recommended his patients should drink solarized water charged with coloured and filtered light. Many thought him a miracle worker, as he would frequently treat the most stubborn ailments with success.

Dinshah Ghadiali, a scientist who was born in India in 1873, devised a complete system of healing involving colour. He proposed that sound, coloured light, magnetism and heat were all different frequencies of one single energy. He correlated colour and other vibrations directly to specific areas of the body and its functions. In 1939 he published his theories in *The Spectro-Chrome Metry Encyclopedia*. He proposed that just as every chemical substance showed a unique spectral analysis, which means that each substance absorbs and reflects different frequencies of light energy, so the body would absorb and reflect colours depending on its state of health. Ghadiali also devised a machine that projected colour.

At the beginning of the 20th century in the USA, optometrist Dr Harry R. Spitter developed a colour healing system he called syntonics. He founded the College of Syntonic Optometry in 1933, where he

▽ **Transparent coloured filters are an important tool in colour therapy that can be used to carry specific energies.**

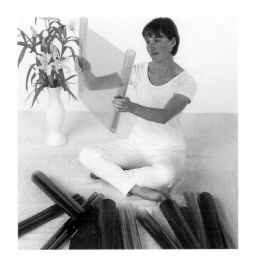

taught that light shone through precise combinations of 31 colour filters directly into the eyes could have profound healing effects on many aspects of the glandular and nervous systems, as well as significantly improving vision. Spitter's work was continued and developed after his death by Jacob Liberman, who uses a system of 20 coloured filters in holistic healing.

The use of colour and light as healing tools faded into the background as the use of new drugs became more widespread. Pharmaceutical drugs became available to treat conditions where sunlight and fresh air had been recommended. As more drugs arrived, the knowledge of utilizing light, colour and other natural resources to heal was no longer used. Recently, the popularity of colour and light as healing tools has increased, particularly as the limits of pharmacology and the complex difficulties of certain diseases are being recognized.

Colour essences

Many of the pioneers of colour healing found that their patients benefited from drinking water charged with natural sunlight or specific wavelengths of colour. Some theorized that the atomic structure of the water was somehow altered and given particular life-enhancing properties. These theories hold renewed interest for scientists today. Medical researchers are currently investigating techniques to target specific light frequencies on diseased tissue to restore normal functioning to the cells.

Colour essences are regaining popularity as vibrational healers. They contain nothing other than water that has been subtly energized and altered by the action of natural sunlight through a coloured filter.

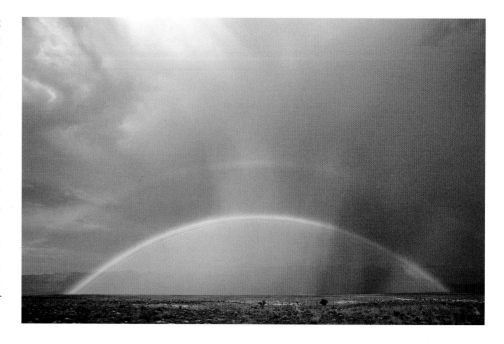

△ The purity of single coloured light that is shown in a rainbow is what makes colour essences such a powerful healing tool.

▽ Medieval doctors would often use the early morning dew gathered from flowers, knowing that it possessed unique balancing properties.

They are easy to make and, like all vibrational remedies, have the advantage of being self-regulating. This means that the body will only make use of the energy within the essence if it is appropriate. Vibrational healing seems to work by reminding the body of its natural state of balance, which it needs to return to after some stress or shock.

Although simple to make, colour essences can be effective tools for healing. Rapid release of stress can sometimes feel uncomfortable. If this is experienced, simply reduce or stop using the essence for a day or two. Taking essences last thing at night and immediately on waking is a good way to bring a person back to a state of balance.

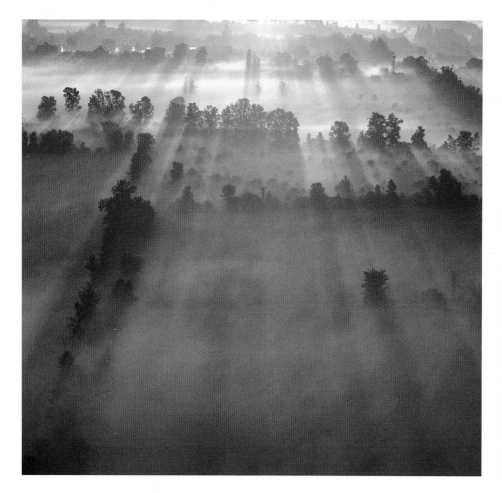

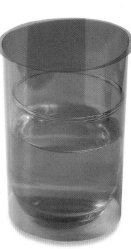

▷ Water can be charged with a colour using sunlight. Take a glass of water and surround it with a coloured gel and cut a disc from another piece to cover the top. Make sure the glass is surrounded then leave it in direct sunlight for two hours.

TO MAKE A VIBRATIONAL ESSENCE

You will need:

1. Clean drinking water, spring water or mineral water is best

2. A plain glass container

3. Colour gels from theatrical lighting suppliers or other coloured filters

4. Brown glass storage bottles

5. Labels

6. A preservative, such as alcohol, cider vinegar or vegetable glycerine

method

1. Pour the water into the glass vessel. Stand it on a colour filter of your choice and cover it with another filter in the same colour. (Colour gels can be made into cones or laid across the top of the vessel.) Leave the vessel in bright natural sunlight for at least two hours.

2. If you are going to keep the essence for future use it will need to be bottled – preferably in brown (neutral amber) glass to reduce exposure to light.

3. It is a good idea to add a preservative to your essence to keep it stable unless you are going to use it immediately. A 50/50 mix of energized water and alcohol such as brandy or vodka will keep

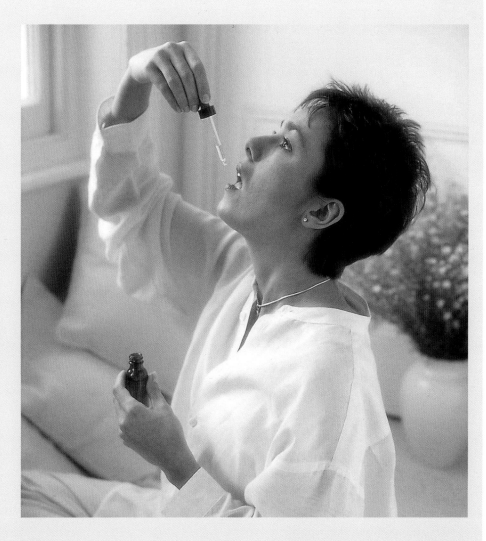

for many months. Cider vinegar, honey or vegetable glycerine can also be used as preservatives if you can't use alcohol.

uses

1. A little can be drunk each day in water. If kept in a dropper bottle, the essence can be taken as and when you need it, either directly dropped into the mouth or mixed with a little water.

2. Drops can be placed straight on to pulse points at the wrists, side of the neck or on the forehead.

3. Add colour essence to a diffuser sprayer filled with water. Spray around the room or around the body for immediate effect.

4. Rub a drop or two on to the area needing help, or the related chakra point.

5. A drop or two can be added to bath water or massage oil.

6. A few drops can be added to water in an oil burner, with or without the additions of essential oils.

△ Taking a few drops of a colour essence three or four times a day can quickly restore balanced energy.

▽ Rubbing a drop of essence into an area of imbalance can speed up the healing process.

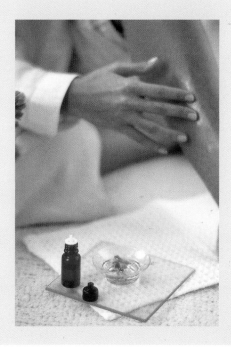

▽ Using a diffuser spray with water and a couple of drops of essence can quickly bring a colour vibration to a whole space.

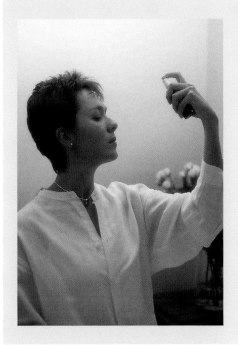

Plants and colour

All over the world plants have been used to help keep the body healthy and to fight disease. Today, herbalism is still the most practical source of healthcare for a majority of the planet's population. Many of the herbs that are in common use indicate by their colour, shape, habit and popular associations how they can be used in healing. The name given to this information is the Doctrine of Signatures, and it has been used as a guide to healers for centuries.

HEALING FLOWERS

Two types of yellow flowers are particularly powerful healing plants. Yellow helps release tension, boosting optimism and relaxation.

St John's wort (*Hypericum perforatum*) is a roadside plant that in midsummer produces a head of bright yellow flowers. This suggests that it acts on the upper abdomen and, through its complementary colour violet, on the brain. In recent years St John's wort has been used as a treatment for depression and for lightening heavy moods. When extracted, the essential oil of the plant is a rich deep red, which can be helpful in boosting energy and the immune system.

The familiar dandelion (*Taraxacum officinale*) is another yellow flower with a wealth of healing properties. Its leaves and root are two of the best known liver tonics and diuretics. Leaves can be eaten in salads and the roasted root makes a coffee substitute. Dandelion flower essence and oil are wonderfully effective muscle relaxants that also help release rigid mental belief systems. The way the seed heads disperse at the slightest breeze is seen as a signature for the quality of letting go.

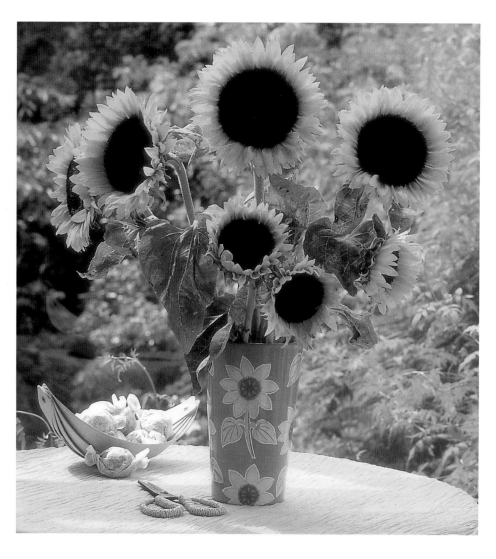

△ The sunflower is sacred to the sun in its native Mexico, and its seeds have been used to treat cold, damp illnesses such as coughs and colds.

▷ Flower essences are a simple way to use plants' energetic and vibrational properties.

flower essences

Paracelsus, the 16th-century Swiss physician and occultist, is believed to have used the dew of flowers for his healing practice and there is some evidence that flower waters were also an integral part of Tibetan medical practices.

Early in the 20th century the gifted homeopath Dr Edward Bach made his own important discoveries about the healing properties of flower essences. He energized

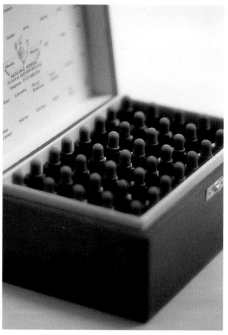

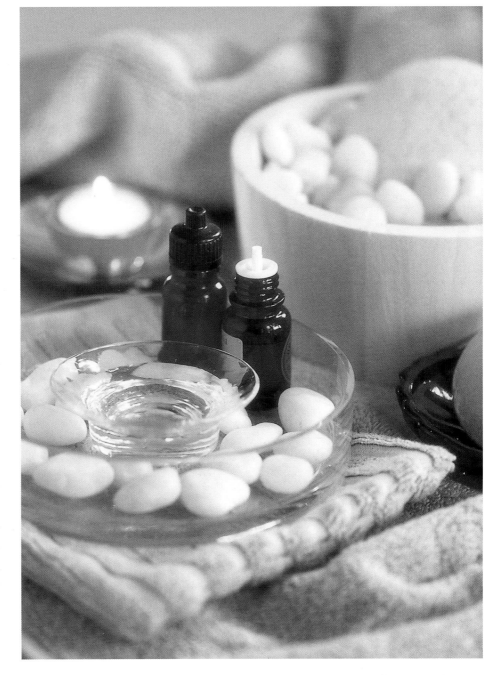

▷ Essential oils are made from the concentrated extracts of plants. They can often be linked to colour energies and used alongside other colour healing techniques.

water with sunlight and flowers or other plant parts to create a set of 38 remedies. They were designed to rebalance the emotional disharmony that Bach saw as underlying all diseases. Dr Bach was often drawn to choose his remedies by the colour as well as other qualities of the plant. Flower essences are now made all around the world to help people bring balance into their lives, and colour plays an important part in explaining how they work.

energizing flowers

Red flowers often boost energy levels, for example, scarlet pimpernel (*Anagallis arvensis*) is a bright red, ground hugging plant whose flowers open only in sunshine. It used to be a popular remedy for heavy moods and depression, but today the flower essence of scarlet pimpernel is more often employed to energize and clear deep-seated blocks. The elm tree has tiny deep red and purple flowers, and their flower essence helps to clear the body and mind when

▽ Red coloured plants and flowers often have rich, heady perfumes that can be sensual, energizing and grounding.

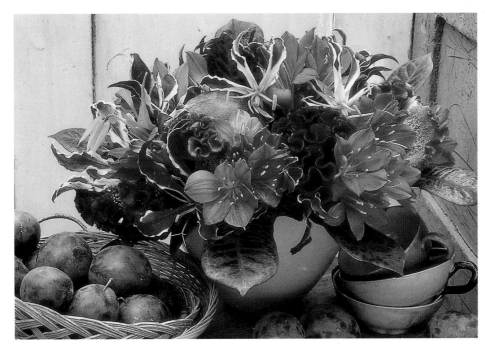

fatigue and confusion have set in. Here the red stimulates the energy reserves and the purple balances the mind.

calming flowers

Blue flowers will often bring a sense of peace and help with communication and expression. Forget-me-not (*Myosotis arvensis*) can aid memory and help those who feel isolated and cut off from deeper levels of experience. Sage (*Salvia officinalis*) has violet-blue flowers that suggest it will be effective in the areas of the head and throat, and the leaves make an antiseptic gargle. The essential oil used very sparingly can help with certain types of headache. The flower essence helps to give a broader outlook on life and balances the mind.

Colour and crystals

Ancient Ayurvedic texts that describe the traditional healing techniques of India speak of seven rays of light that shone from the creator to make the solar system. These rainbow colours are said to nourish the seven planets, which in turn activate the gemstones found within the earth. According to the Ayurveda, gemstones radiate their energy out into their surroundings and, if they are worn, they bring the influence of their light into the wearer's life.

As in many traditional systems of healing there is a close correlation between the colour of gemstones and their healing properties. Once the key concepts for each colour are recognized, it is easy to identify how a crystal or gemstone will bring the qualities of its planet to interact with our personal energy. For example, red is the colour of Mars, so red stones are used to enhance Martian qualities like courage,

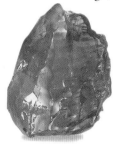

▷ **Transparent crystals, like this orange calcite, allow the passage of sunlight right through the unique atomic structure of the rock.**

▽ **The endless range of coloured minerals and crystals make them an ideal way to introduce colour into a healing session.**

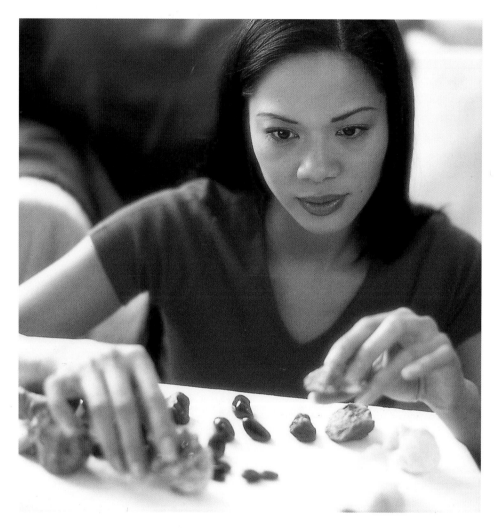

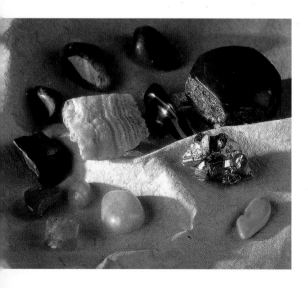

△ **Colour selection can be made using a group of different coloured crystals. Simply notice which stones attract the eye as you gaze over them.**

strength and protection. Green is the colour of Venus, and green stones help with relationships and creativity.

The colour of a crystal affects us in two ways – through our eyes and by its placement on the body. Crystals are coherent, organized forms of matter and the colour they transmit is a focused, powerful vibration. Crystals that are transparent, letting light right through them, will generally have a more pronounced and focused effect than opaque stones, where the light frequencies are both absorbed and radiated outwards in a more diffuse manner.

warm coloured stones

Red stones will be energizing and stimulating. Rich, bright reds, such as garnet, ruby and zircon, can be quite dramatic in their effects. The opaque or tawny reds of jasper and iron quartz create a more grounded, practical energy.

Orange stones are excellent for use in situations of shock and trauma. They will energize the repair mechanisms within the body. Carnelian and orange calcite will soothe and restore, while topaz and rutilated quartz help to strengthen and reintegrate dissipated energies.

Yellow stones support the sense of self, energizing the solar plexus and so reducing tension and anxiety. Citrine, yellow fluorite, tiger's eye and amber create clarity, awareness and confidence.

cool coloured stones

Green stones balance the heart, calm the emotions and stimulate personal potential for growth. Green aventurine and green tourmaline are good emotional stabilizers. Emerald and moss agate encourage harmony with our surroundings. Malachite, dioptase and peridot help to release emotional pain.

Light blue stones support communication skills and work well to strengthen the immune system. Turquoise and aquamarine encourage flexibility and support the subtle energy systems of the body. Blue lace agate and celestite release tensions and lift heavy moods.

Dark blue stones such as lapis lazuli, sodalite, sapphire and kyanite quieten the normal thought processes and encourage intuition. They can also help to release long-held stresses, encouraging deep peace.

Violet stones, such as amethyst, fluorite and sugilite, make excellent objects for meditation and contemplation. They encourage the integration of all aspects of the self.

▽ **Green and turquoise stones help to calm the emotions and enhance subtle perceptions and psychic skills.**

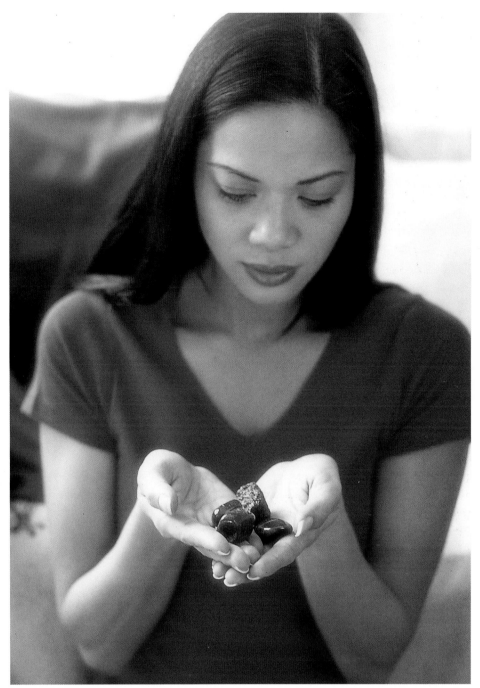

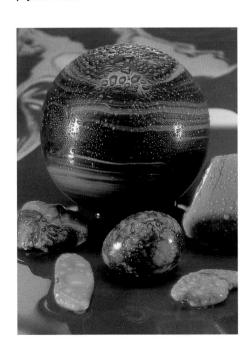

crystals of other colours

White and clear stones generally amplify the life-sustaining energies of the body. They bring clarity, purification, orderliness and harmony. Clear quartz, calcite and selenite energize, while moonstone, milky quartz and other translucent white or cloudy stones have a soothing, gently cleansing effect.

Black stones – obsidian, smoky quartz, black tourmaline and haematite – can help to release deep energy imbalances. They focus awareness inwards, calming the body and mind by speeding the release of unwanted energies.

Pink stones are useful for releasing emotional tension and helping to improve self-confidence and acceptance. Rose quartz,

△ **Peace and quiet can be quickly experienced just by holding or gazing at a blue stone. Colour and natural crystal energy combine to great effect.**

rhodocrosite, rhodonite and kunzite remove the stresses that prevent us from being at ease in the world and can be helpful in countering aggressive situations.

Any crystal, if you are drawn to it, will have a healing effect. If you want one to help you with a specific problem, look at a collection of different stones and work with those you are attracted to. The colour correspondences of the crystals can indicate the root of the difficulty or may give you some clues to other steps you can take to enhance your health and wellbeing.

Double colour healing

Single colours are very effective healing and assessment tools. However, if two colours are used in combination, both the healing and the assessment capacities increase. In the last 30 years three systems have developed that make use of the double-colour technique for healing – AuraSoma, AuraLight and AvaTara. All consist of coloured oil floating on top of a different coloured water in clear bottles. Cards can also be used as double-colour healing and assessment tools. They may have windows of theatrical spotlight gels or stained glass, or be simply printed with blocks of colour.

With all colour combinations, the top colour represents the conscious, the present and the most apparent energies. The lower colour represents the underlying factors, the past or roots of the situation and associated unconscious issues.

how to use a double-colour system

As with single colour selection, just pick the combination that appeals to you most. Your choice will reflect your current situation. Each of the colours is then interpreted through its correspondences. Try also selecting the combination you like the least, as this will reflect areas that may need a different kind of attention.

Sometimes several combinations may be chosen. The first choice can represent the roots of the present situation, the second choice can indicate the difficulties encountered, and the third choice can show the primary healing requirements.

▽ **Colour rarely appears isolated in nature. Combinations of colour build up complex and specific effects, affecting moods and thoughts.**

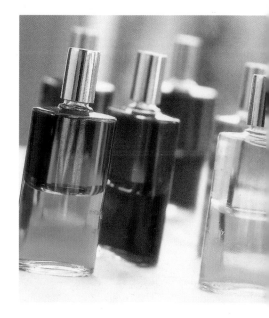

△ **Bottles of dual-coloured liquid capture the attention easily, regardless of any understanding of colour healing.**

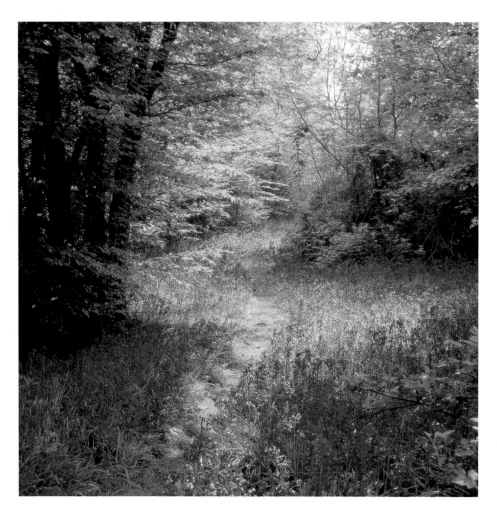

examples of double-colour selection

Choice 1 – yellow over red – the roots of the situation

• Physically this could indicate the possibility of tension or digestive difficulties (yellow) with a need for activity or initiative (red).

• Emotionally this may show that fear or anxiety (yellow) is being fed by anger or passion (red).

• Mentally, there is a need for clear, logical choices (yellow) to begin new projects (red).

• Spiritually there may be a need to get to know yourself better (yellow) in order to become more secure and grounded in the world (red).

choice 2 – green over blue – the difficulties encountered

• Physically there may be breathing problems (green), and some communication difficulties (blue).

• Emotionally, there might be a feeling of being confined (green) by ideas and beliefs (blue).

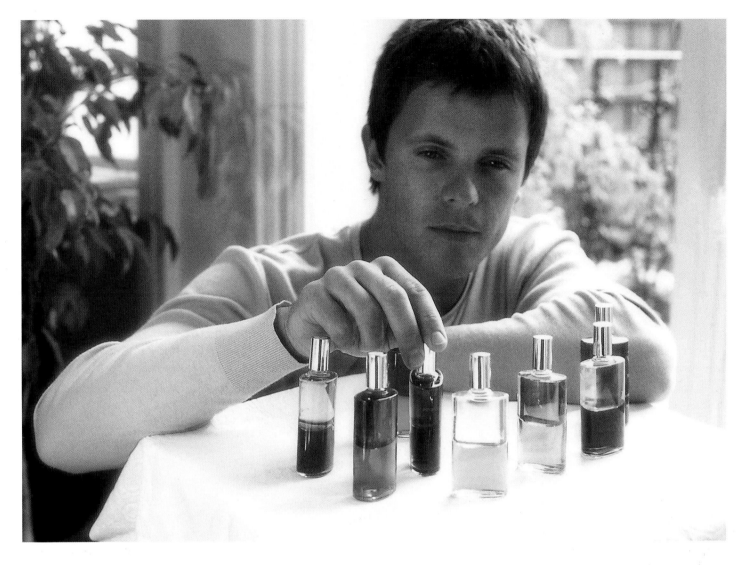

• Mentally, there is a definite need for space (green) to find peace (blue).

• Spiritually, there is a desire to go your own way (green) in a natural flow (blue).

choice 3 – violet over turquoise – primary healing requirements

• Physically, there is a need to be in quiet and harmonious surroundings (violet) so

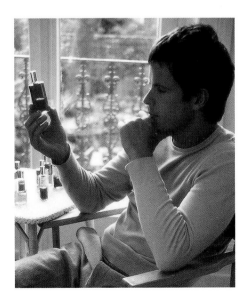

that you can settle down and just be yourself (turquoise)

• Emotionally, consider cutting away illusion and delusion (violet) to find where the truth is for you (turquoise)

• Mentally, you need to gain inspiration (violet) from your own resources (turquoise)

• Spiritually, there is a need to heal yourself in order to feel at one with life (violet) and be able to express yourself freely (turquoise)

how double colours can heal

In a healing situation, once the choices have been made and discussed, issues often rise to the surface. Colour has a habit of bringing to the attention facets of life that have remained hidden. This gives an opportunity for healing. One way to bring healing is to have contact with the chosen combinations for a few minutes. If bottles are being used, they can be held or placed around the body.

◁ **Your choices can be held up to the light or close to the body, for the healing effect of colour to be absorbed.**

△ **Selection from a range of double-colours elicits deep levels of information about a person's needs and direction in life. The choice of bottle will be made on an intuitive level.**

The oil and water constituents of the bottles can also be massaged into the hands, feet or other appropriate places. If the combination is a light gel, it can be projected on to the body, or on to a wall to be looked at. The constituents of the combinations can also be introduced through diet, lifestyle or through your surroundings.

In the third example given here, the primary requirements were shown to be violet over turquoise. This could suggest spending quiet periods alone, and also introducing violet and turquoise items temporarily into the living space. Wearing two of the appropriate colours can be an immediate way to bring those energies into your life. This could be through single coloured separates or by wearing ties or scarves of the colours. Even such simple changes can have profound effects.

Colour and shape

Philosophers and mystics have always been interested in exploring the origins of creation. Eastern and Western thinkers have traditionally used light and colour combined with geometric shapes to help define the forces of the universe in symbolic terms.

sacred shapes

The science of geometry is the basic patterning of all matter in creation. In Classical Greece the philosopher Plato devised a system of representing the elements with coloured geometric forms, in an attempt to explain the building blocks of all existence, including spiritual realities. Platonic Solids define how to form physical matter, because they represent the only way atoms can pack together. Like the elements and colours,

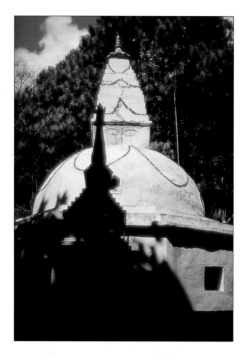

energy interacts to form physical matter. The Platonic Solids, therefore, encapsulate our understanding of the universe.

At around the same time that Plato was working, Indian philosophers were also choosing different shapes and colours to represent the elements. They called the elements and their symbols tattvas, literally: those things that possess distinction.

Shape holds and defines colour, giving it solidity and presence, while colour imparts different qualities to shape. A viewer reacts differently to a blue triangle and a red triangle. A yellow circle feels different to a yellow square. The human brain's response to various stimuli has allowed the non-verbal language of symbolism to develop in every culture.

▽ **A set of Platonic Solids cut out of clear quartz: (left to right) cube of Earth; octahedron of Air; tetrahedron of Fire; dodecahedron of Ether; and icosahedron of Water.**

△ **Shape as well as colour contains specific energies. These are harnessed especially in religious buildings to enhance the spiritual qualities of the surroundings.**

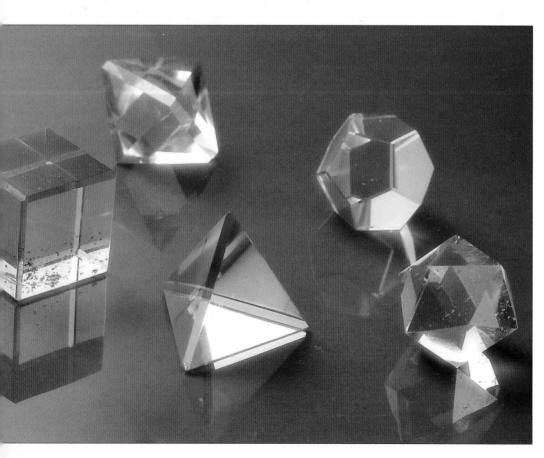

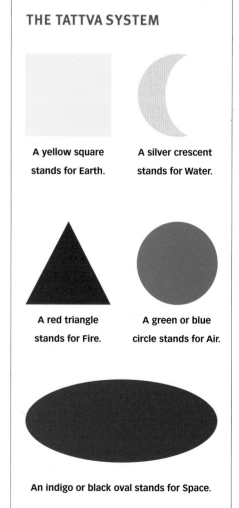

THE TATTVA SYSTEM

A yellow square stands for Earth.

A silver crescent stands for Water.

A red triangle stands for Fire.

A green or blue circle stands for Air.

An indigo or black oval stands for Space.

Colour therapists such as Theo Gimbel and Howard and Dorothy Sun have introduced shape into their colour healing work. Theo Gimbel shines coloured light through shaped apertures on to the body to help restore balance to its subtle energy systems. The Suns assess their patients' wellbeing after asking them to choose from a range of coloured shapes based on the Platonic solids. This gives an accurate profile of both personality and situation. Similar assessment techniques are continuing to be developed as it becomes more widely understood that our instinctive choices of colour and shape can accurately indicate underlying factors in our lives.

Mary Hykel Hunt, a Welsh psychologist and colour worker, is in a unique position

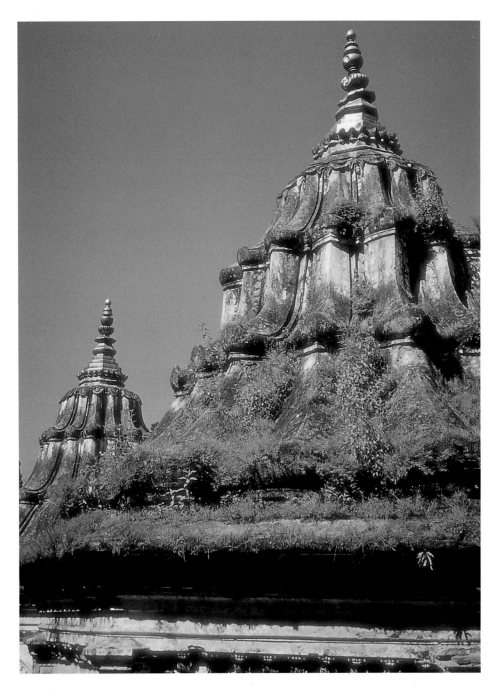

△ **The forms of classical Indian architecture are precisely proportioned to reflect the elemental shapes of the tattvas, such as the crescent, square, cone and sphere.**

WHAT'S IN A NAME?

Ask a friend, colleague or family member if you can look at their name for colours and shapes. Sit quietly, thinking about the name, and intuit what colours and shapes seem to be present in it.

Let us imagine that the name you're thinking about is Kathy. You might feel that the name is made up of a three-dimensional blue rectangle (or double cube) followed by a red circle, a brown cube and a yellow crescent.

The three-dimensional rectangle or double cube represents Earth, coloured with the blue of communication. It suggests someone with practical communication skills. The cube again represents Earth, this time coloured brown for practicality and focus. This shows creative and nurturing skills put to practical use.

The circle represents Air, coloured red for activity. This activates or energizes communication.

The crescent represents Water, coloured yellow to show thought processes, anxiety and joy. This hints at the emotions that lie behind the practical activity, and suggests that there may be some problems with self-criticism.

to explore the relationship between shape, colour and personality. From birth she has been synaesthetic, that is, her senses of sight and sound are combined so that she experiences colour and shape with each sound she hears. This has enabled Hykel Hunt to train others to explore the innate ability we all have of translating one sense into another. Hykel Hunt's workshops provide people with a whole series of symbols, similar to the tattvas, with which to intuitively explore the energy make-up of the world around them.

People's names provide a rich source of intuitive exploration. Hykel Hunt teaches how to intuit coloured shapes from the sound of someone's name and then to use those colours and shapes to discover the

skills and gifts of that person. The more you try to link colour, shape and sound, the more successful and confident you will become. Try the name visualization exercise in a group of people, and you will find remarkably similar results.

This suggests that people can successfully tap into their innate skills with a little practice and encouragement. It also backs up the findings of the Indian and Greek philosophers, who saw correlations and correspondences between colour, shape and human experience.

The life-supporting chakras

The chakra system is one of the most well-known systems of annotating human subtle energies, and has been adopted from the ancient Vedic tradition of India. The chakra system describes a series of large energy vortices aligned to the spine and numerous smaller ones throughout the body. In classical texts many correspondences were allocated to each chakra, like shape, animals, colours and deities, to describe the energies and qualities present.

As healers and spiritual workers in the West have became more familiar with the chakras, they, too, have allocated colours to each chakra from the rainbow of visible light. This arrangement of colours and chakras is easy to remember and the correlation between chakras and colours works well. The colours given in the Vedic texts are different for some chakras, adding an extra dimension to understanding how the chakras work.

The chakras could be divided into two sections. Those supporting life physically, and reflecting our connection to the world, correspond to the western colours; red, orange and yellow. The chakras where we relate to the world and through which we express our individuality correspond to green, blue and violet. The precision of yoga postures allows them to be related to the chakras and the different colour energies. Each yoga posture can be seen to activate one or more chakra, bringing in the corresponding colours.

▽ **Preparing to enter the yoga posture known as the Warrior. This posture reflects the martial quality of the red energy.**

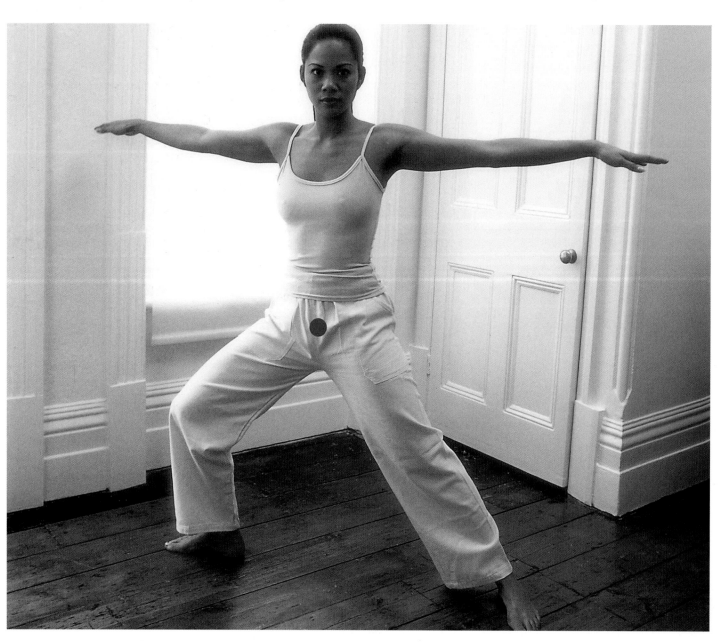

the root chakra

The base or root chakra is located at the base of the spine. Physically this is linked to the adrenal glands which supply the hormones that provide the fright and flight mechanism for survival. It governs the hip and legs as a means to move and our connection to the planet. This aligns to red in Western traditions, or yellow in the Vedic traditions, relating to the earth element.

The wide-stride yoga positions work directly on the root chakra. Holding these positions, even if just for a few seconds, brings an increase in bloodflow, warmth and the invigorating qualities of red.

the sacral chakra

The sacral chakra is located midway between the navel and the pubic bone, and is related to the sacrum area of the spine.

▽ **Most people find this position eases lower back problems as well as helping all the organs in the lower areas of the abdomen.**

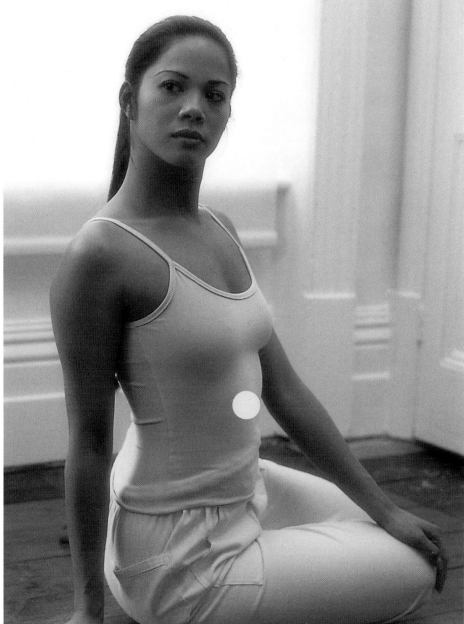

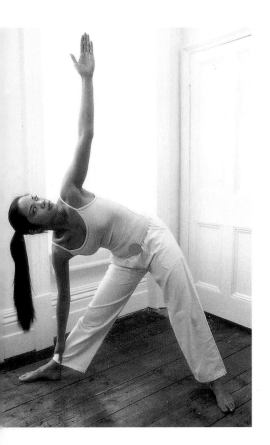

△ **A simple twist of the trunk of the body has the added benefit of toning the waist muscles.**

Associated with the reproductive organs, the sacral chakra deals with creativity on all levels. The large intestine is also situated here, emphasising the need to release unwanted energies from the body. Orange also deals with all these qualities and the Vedic colour of the sacral chakra is white, emphasising the cleansing and clearing needed to keep this chakra in a healthy flow of energy.

The yoga position called the Triangle releases tension from the sacrum, stimulating bloodflow to the large intestine and lower pelvis. It brings orange energy into the lower abdomen, releasing any energy blocks or stress.

the solar plexus chakra

The third chakra, or the solar plexus, is located between the bottom of the ribcage and the navel. It is linked to the lumbar spine and the pancreas. In the Western tradition yellow is related to this chakra, as digestion and assimilation of energy physically, emotionally and mentally are crucial for people to harness their personal power. However, in the Vedic tradition, the colour red is allocated to this chakra as it underlines the fiery nature of digestion that is needed to sustain our bodies.

Any activity that creates a twist in the lumbar region of the spine increases the amount of yellow energy available to the body. It also tones the internal organs of the upper abdomen and increases the flexibility of the spine.

The chakras of individual expression

When the classical Vedic texts were translated and brought to the West, they arrived at a time when the physical functions of the body associated with the root and sacral chakras were shunned by society. This attitude persisted in the subsequent spiritual writings of the Western teachers, which exhorted the focus of the development of the heart, throat, brow and crown chakras. It has only been in recent years that this attitude has been dropped in the recognition that without the support of the other chakras, there is no means to sustain practical expression of spirituality. Subsequently, the colours associated with the upper-body chakras (green, blue, indigo, violet and white) were thought to be more spiritual than the red, orange and yellows of the root, sacral and solar plexus chakras. For health and well-being we need all our chakras and all colours, for only with access to the full spectrum, can we reach our full potential.

the heart chakra

The heart chakra is located at the centre of the chest. It is linked to the thoracic vertebrae that run from the neck down to the base of the ribs. The chakra is related to the thymus gland, the heart, lungs and the arms. In both of the colour systems, this chakra is green, the colour midway in the rainbow spectrum and chakra system, thus showing its importance for balancing our lives.

Yoga positions that open and stretch the ribcage and shoulders introduce more green energy into the body. The idea with a posture like the Cobra, shown here, is to keep the shoulders as relaxed as possible while maintaining the position.

the throat chakra

This chakra is related to the cervical vertebrae of the neck. The glands linked to this chakra are the thyroid and parathyroids that control the rate of metabolism. The ears, nose and mouth are also under the influence of this chakra which also deals with communication and expression of an individual's creativity. This is not necessarily just through speech, but the use of any form of communication. This chakra is associated with blue in both colour systems.

Yoga poses that increase the flow of blue energy involve flexion and extension of the neck. This encourages the increase of all energy flows between the head and torso.

the brow chakra

The sixth chakra is known as the brow chakra or the Third Eye. It is related to the pineal gland situated in the centre of the

▽ **Green energy is linked to the act of breathing. It is easy to mistakenly hold the breath while doing the Cobra, rather than relaxing and breathing deeply. Focusing the eyes of the brow chakra brings in blue and indigo energy.**

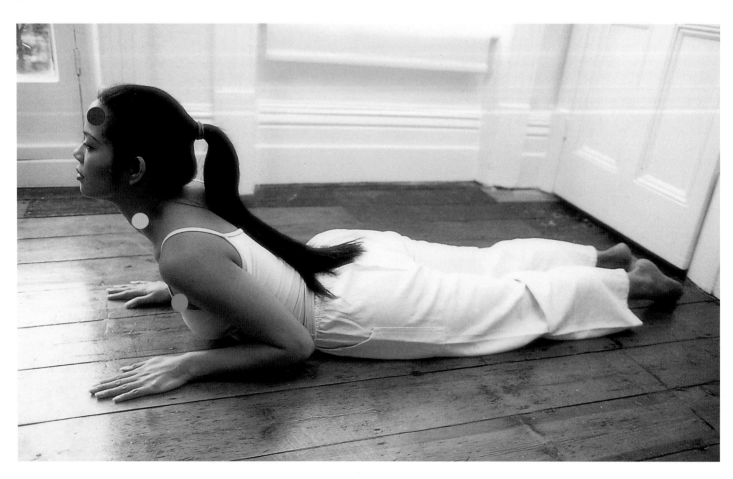

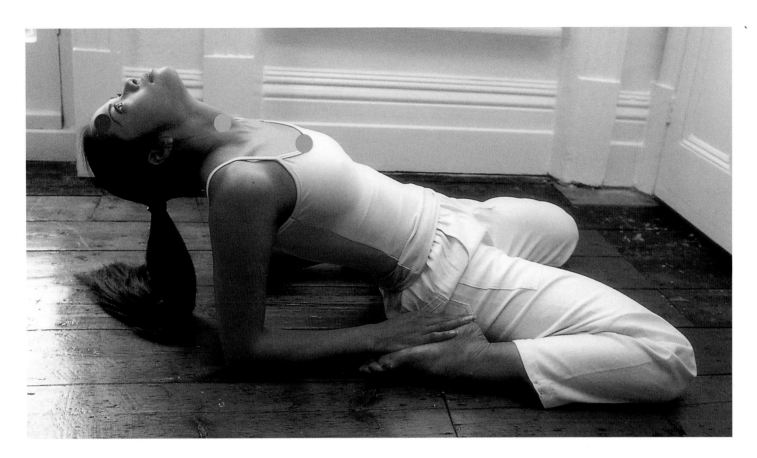

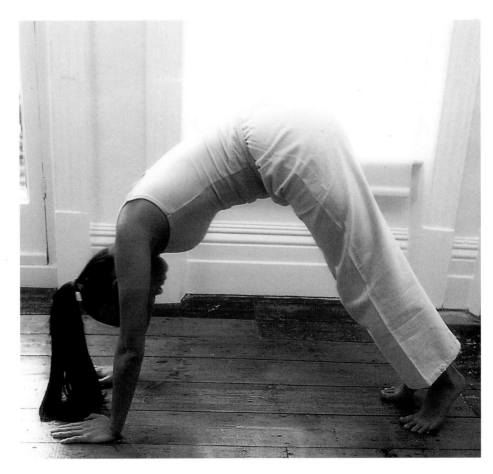

△ **This pose is a combination of both the Camel position and the Fish position. Here the neck is moved gently and slowly without jerking or any sudden movement.**

head. This gland maintains the daily cycles of activity and moods through a series of complex hormones, melatonin and sera-tonin. It is said that this chakra can remain at a low level of activity for many people. It relates to indigo or midnight blue, cor-responding to intuition and imagination.

The yoga pose, a variation of both the Camel and the Fish, brings indigo energy into the body. From a lying position, the back is arched, supported by the elbows. The neck is relaxed and the head allowed to fall back towards the floor. The body returns to lying down on release.

the crown chakra

This chakra, or thousand-petalled lotus as it is sometimes known, is situated above crown of the head. It is linked to all other chakras and to the whole of the individual. It correlates to violet, white and gold, but

is sometimes related to the whole rainbow spectrum. The gland associated with the crown is usually the pituitary, but some texts alternate this with the pineal. The pituitary is the master-controlling gland for the whole body and ensures the distribution of

information as chemical messengers. The traditional yoga pose here is the Headstand, but for most people the Dog pose works well. This concentrates violet energy in the head, helping the functions of the brain to harmonise and integrate.

▷ **This pose allows you to stretch your back like a cat or dog does when they wake up. The violet energy quietens you if you want to sleep, or enlivens you if you want to be more awake.**

Colour visualization

In Tibetan meditation practices, different aspects of energy are visualized as spheres of coloured light. Visual imagery of many sorts is a major part of Tibetan spiritual techniques, along with the use of breath control, sound and posture.

Complex visualizations take practice to achieve, but the focus required is itself of benefit, by taking the mind away from everyday concerns. In all visualization exercises it is important to remember that cinema-like clarity and detail are not necessary to achieve success. Simply reading through an exercise begins to create the right emotional picture.

energy sphere visualization

The following exercise is designed to integrate the inner and outer worlds by bringing the colours of the directions into the heart. This leads to a balance of harmony

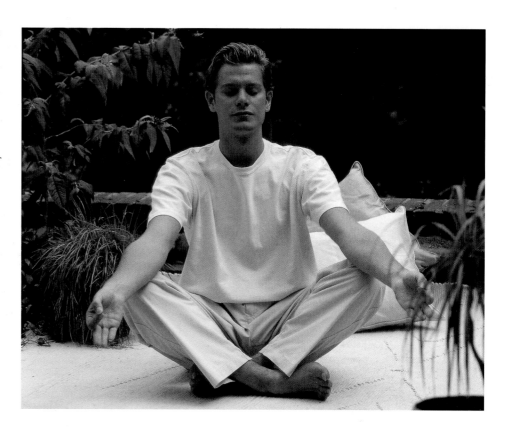

△ **Visualization is the natural function of the human mind to think in pictures.**

with one's surroundings and restores equilibrium in the body, mind and emotions.

1. Sit in a comfortable position, facing the east. Imagine a deep blue lotus with four petals resting at its centre.

2. In the heart of the flower is a luminous clear sphere of light, like crystal. It reflects the blue of the petals and represents the element of space (ether).

3. Before the lotus is a yellow sphere, representing the east, the earth element.

4. To your left, the north, is a green sphere, the air element.

5. Behind you is a red sphere of the west, the fire element.

6. To the right of you is a blue sphere of the south, the water element.

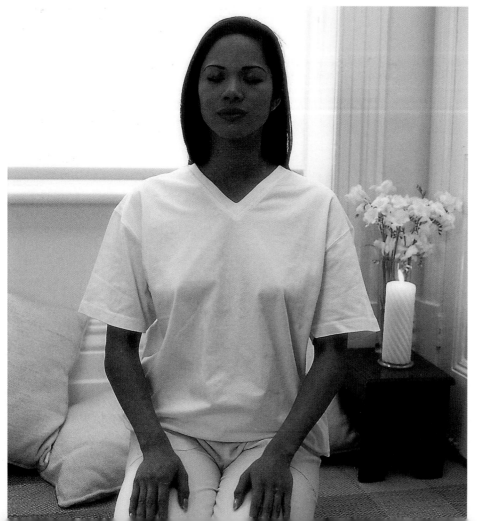

◁ **Visualizing specific colours around you, in the compass directions, then visualizing blue and white flowing through you, is exceptionally relaxing and healing.**

rainbow breathing

This is a simple but effective way of bringing colour energies into your body to restore balance when there has been stress, or to identify which colour energies you are most in need of absorbing.

1. Take a minute to relax and calm your mind with your eyes closed.

2. Imagine the air around you is a rich, deep red. As you breathe in, your whole body fills with red energy. Continue breathing in the red light until you feel you have sufficient, then breathe out the red light through your feet or your spine, into the earth.

3. Next, imagine the air becomes a vibrant, warm orange colour. Breathe in the orange energy in the same way. When you have

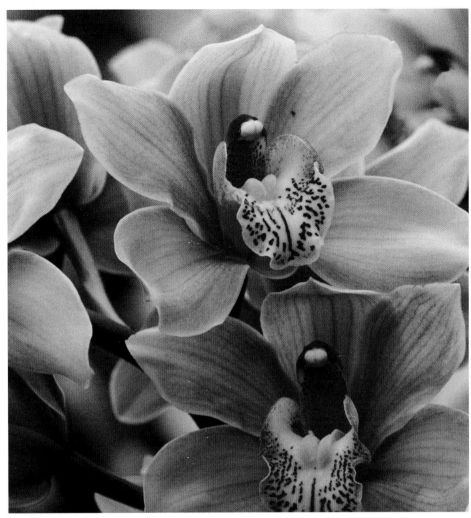

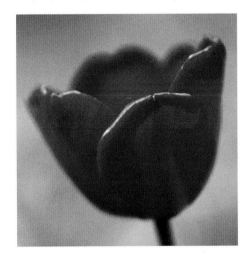

△▽ **Imagining an object of the same colour as the one you are visualizing will help to create a clearer image. Look at a bright coloured flower and imagine yourself breathing in the colour.**

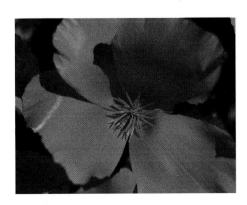

completed the process and breathed it out to the earth, continue with the other colours of the spectrum: yellow, green, blue, indigo and violet.

If you have need for a particular colour energy, concentrate on that visualization and take notice of how it seems to move around the body. Make sure the light goes to every part of your body by paying attention to areas that are difficult to visualize.

protecting the heart of all things

This is a visualization exercise that is extremely valuable when we face difficult circumstances in our lives. It helps to remove fear, which is the cause of all other negative reactions, both from ourselves and from the people around us. Doing this exercise can also help to reduce anger, aggression, irritation and misunderstanding.

1. Right at the centre of your heart chakra, in the middle of your chest, imagine a spark of bright pink light.

2. Keep your imagination on that spark of

△ **The visualization of pink light has a calming, integrating and healing effect on yourself and your surroundings.**

light strong and gradually see it radiating out through the body in a strong pink glow.

3. The spark of pink energy is like a sun in your heart and its light completely fills your body and then continues to expand outwards in a pink halo of light surrounding everything around you.

4. As it touches others, the pink star at their own heart sparks into life, so that the pink energy gets stronger the more people around you it contacts.

5. At the end of the visualization, allow your attention to return to the pink star at your heart, as the surrounding colour fades gently away.

If when you begin the visualization, you see a different colour, allow that to be your focus. It may be more appropriate to the energy of the situation you find yourself in, even if you feel the colours you see to be negative or hostile.

Colour in meditation

Colour is a very powerful tool in all meditation exercises because it has a profound effect on the nervous system, no matter what else may be happening on the surface levels of the mind. Here are two meditation exercises that use colour in different ways. When you use them make sure you are sitting or lying in a comfortable position, with no risk of disturbance or distraction.

absorbing the lights of perfection

One of the main practices in Tibetan Buddhism is to visualize a teacher or enlightened being, such as a buddha, and absorb their enlightened qualities into one's own body in the form of coloured light. The nature or form of the visualized being is not as important as the confidence and faith of the meditator. The being represents all those who have taught us, looked after us, and wished us well in our lives.

The following exercise is calming and clarifying and helps to bring the energy of the mind into its natural state of relaxed quietness. It helps to establish a continual connection to your true nature.

1. Sit quietly for a minute or two. Consider all the teachers and spiritual beings who have inspired you with the qualities of clarity, compassion and truth. Visualize their presence in front of you as a glorious bright

▽ **Feel the coloured lights at brow, throat and heart dissolving all negativity and bringing clarity and peace.**

light suffused with translucent rainbow colours. Within the light is a figure representing all the wisdom of the universe.

2. From the forehead of the figure, a clear white beam enters your forehead and fills your body with light, cleansing all heaviness and negativity from your body.

3. Next, from the throat of the figure of light emerges a ray of ruby red, which enters your own throat. From there, it fills your body and cleanses negativity from your senses.

4. Now from the heart of the figure of light flows a ray of shimmering deep blue, entering your own heart and pervading your whole body, clearing away negativity from your mind.

5. As you have shared the purifying colour vibrations from the being of light, you have merged together so that now there is no distinction, no difference between your energy and the clear compassionate light of the universe.

a tattva meditation

Using the tattvic shapes, the traditional Hindu symbols of the elements, can be an effective way to balance personal energies. Many variations are possible but the aim is to absorb the quality of each element and integrate it into the body.

For this meditation you need to focus on each tattva in turn or concentrate on those you feel need more balance. As you visualize the shape within your body, feel your inbreath entering the symbol, charging it with energy. As you breath out imagine it removing imbalance from that area.

Alternatively, you can place a representation of a particular tattva in front of you on a white wall. As you breathe naturally, imagine that you are breathing in the energy of the element represented by the colour and shape.

The yellow square of Earth sits with its base upon the base of the spine. It can be used when energy is low and there is a lack of motivation.

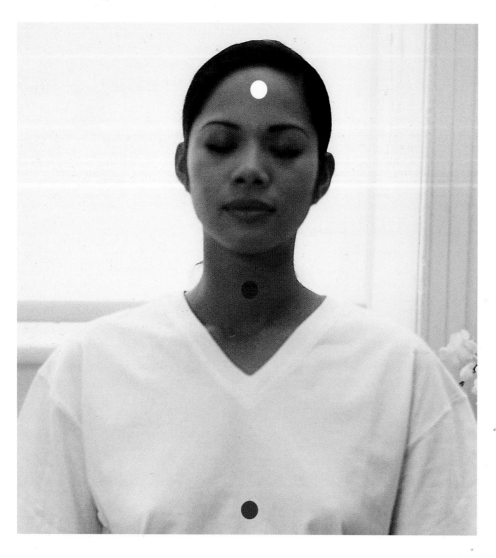

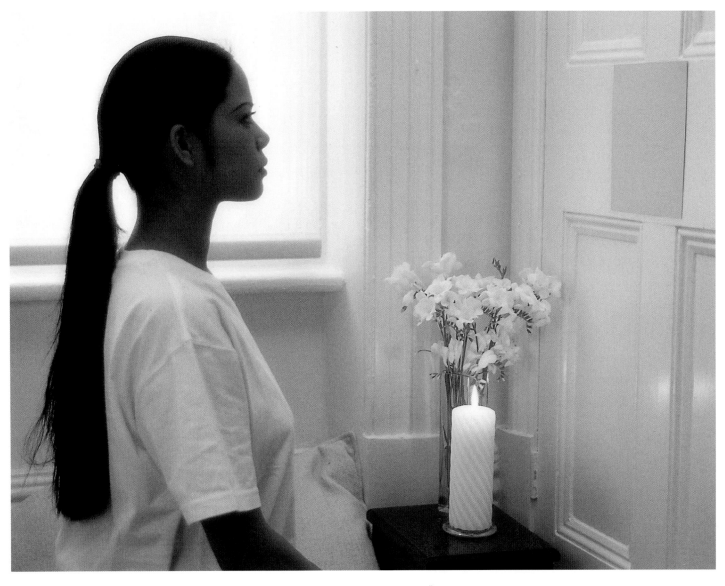

△ Gazing at an elemental tattva shape lets you understand the quality of energy of shape and colour and will balance the element in your body.

▷ Working with coloured shapes on card can be an intuitive way of selecting and balancing your needs at the moment.

The silver-white crescent of the Water element sits between the navel and the pubic bone within the top of the pelvis. Use it when there is indecision, excess of emotion or a feeling of heaviness.

The red triangle of Fire sits pointing downwards from the base of the ribcage towards the navel. It is useful to calm anger, irritation and exhaustion.

The blue circle of Air is in the centre of the chest. It will help focus concentration, reducing agitation and scattered thoughts.

The midnight blue or black egg of Ether or Space sits within the throat. It can soothe feelings of emptiness and uselessness.

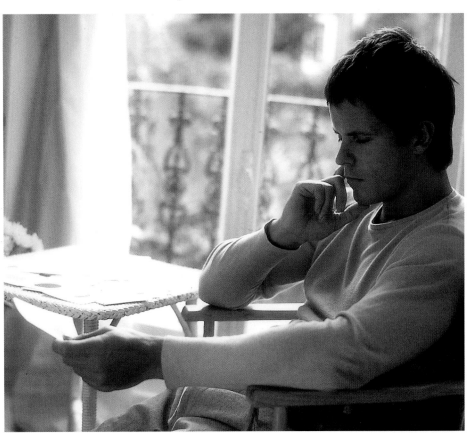

Addresses and Acknowledgements

International Groups

Light Information for Growth and
Healing Trust
(A charitable trust to promote the use of
light, colour and sound in physical,
mental and spiritual health.)
28 Devonshire Road
Bognor Regis
West Sussex PO21 2SY
Email: dorothye.parker@currantbun.com
Web: www.lighttrust.co.uk

International Association of Colour
(A contact for colour therapy schools
worldwide.)
46 Cottenham Road
Histon
Cambridge CB4 9ES

Irlen Institute
(Colour overlays for use in education.)
5380 Village Road
Long Beach CA 90808
USA
Web: www.irlenuk.com

BeColourWise Courses, including
"Name Colour Courses".
Mary Hykel Hunt
Email: hykel@lineone.net

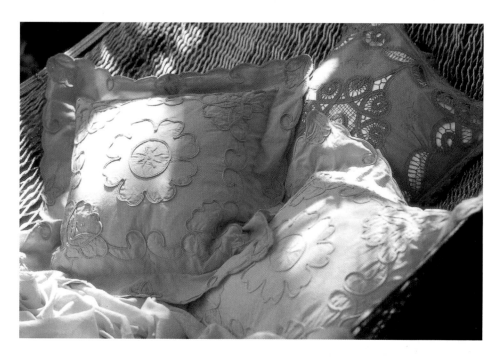

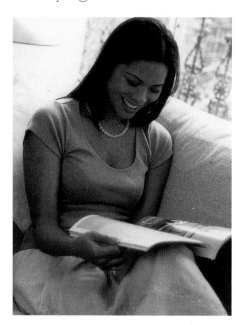

Suppliers

All products are available internationally.
Green Man Essences
PO Box 6
Exminster
Exeter
Devon, EX6 8YE
Suppliers of colour/light essences.
Email: info@greenmanessences.com
Website: www.greenmanessences.com

AuraLight
"Unicornis"
Obi Obi Road
Mapleton QLD 4560
Australia
Manufacturers of two layers of colour
in bottles
Email: info@auralight.net
Web: www.auralight.net

Aura-Soma
Dev Aura
Little London
Tetford
Lincs LN9 6QB
Manufacturers of two layers of colour
in bottles
Email: info@asict.demon.co.uk

AvaTara
Pitt White
Mill Lane
Uplyme
Devon DT7 3TZ
Manufacturers of two layers of colour
in bottles
Email: mail@avataracolour.com
Website: www.avataracolour.com

Acknowledgements

The publishers would like to thank the
following agencies and photographers for
permission to use their images.

AKG 74t; The Art Archive 16bl, 41bl;
David Noble 82b; Elizabeth Whiting
22bl; 26bl; Robert Harding Picture
Library 15tr, 17bl and br, 21b, 23tr, ; The
Ronald Grant Archive 47b; Scala 15bl,
16tr; Sonia Halliday 48ml, and Laura
Lushington 43tl; The Stock Market 13br,
20tr, 21tr, 24bl, 28b, 36t, 44ml, 47tl; Sue
and Simon Lilly 84t, 85; Sylvia Corday
p11br; 12br;17tl; 48tl.

Index

advertising, 20
alcohol, 71
animals, 12, 13
artificial light, 56–7
assessment, single colour, 60–1
AuraLight, 82
AuraSoma, 82
autonomic nervous system, 54, 55
autumn colours, 19
AvaTara, 82
Ayurveda, 80

Babitt, Dr Edwin, 75
Bach, Dr Edward, 78–9
bathrooms, 23
bedrooms, 26
black, 46–7
    crystals, 81
    cultural variations, 14
    meditation, 93
    single colour assessment, 60–1
blue, 40–1
    chakras, 88
    colour visualization, 90
    commercial use of colour, 20–1
    crystals, 81
    double-colour healing, 82–3
    flowers, 79
    foods, 71
    light, 56
    meditation, 93
    single colour assessment, 60–1
brain, 54–5
breathing, rainbow, 91
brow chakra, 88–9
brown, 50, 60–1
Buddhism, 92

camouflage, 13

cells: eyes, 54–5
    plants, 56
chakras, 86–9
choosing colours, 58–9
clothes, 16–17, 18–19
co-ordinating colour, 18–19
colour essences, 76–7
colour healing: chakras, 86–9
    crystals, 80–1
    double-colour healing, 82–3
    essences, 76–7
    plants, 78–9
    shapes, 84–5
    theories, 74–5
colour placement, 62–3
colour vision, 12, 54–5
colour wheel, 18
commercial use of colour, 20–1
complementary colours, 18
cone cells, eyes, 54–5
crown chakra, 89
crystals, 80–1
cultural variations, 14–15

dandelion, 78
death, 14
Doctrine of Signatures, 78
double-colour healing, 82–3
drugs, 75
dyes, 16
dyslexia, 62–3

elements, feng shui, 28–9
endocrine system, 55
energy: chakras, 86
    colour visualization, 90–1
entrance halls, 22–3
environments, natural, 10–11
essences: colour, 76–7
    flower, 78–9
essential oils, 79
examinations, 62
eyes, 12, 54–5

feng shui, 28–9
flowers, 78–9

fluorescent lighting, 57
food, 64–71
food additives, 71
fruit, 66–71

gemstones, 80–1
genetically modified foods, 71
geometry, 84
Ghadiali, Dinshah, 75
Gimbel, Theo, 85
Goethe, J.W. von, 74
gold, single colour assessment, 60–1
Greece, 84, 85
green, 38–9
    chakras, 88
    colour visualization, 90
    commercial use of colour, 21
    crystals, 80, 81
    cultural variations, 15
    double-colour healing, 82–3
    foods, 70
    light, 56
    single colour assessment, 60–1
grey, 51, 60–1

halls, 22–3
heart chakra, 88
herbalism, 78
Hinduism, 92
holidays, 10–11
homes, 22–7
hormones, 55
Hunt, Mary Hykel, 85
hyperactivity, 63
hypothalamus, 54, 55

India, 80, 84, 85, 86
indigo, 42–3
    chakras, 88, 89

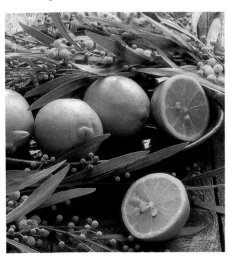

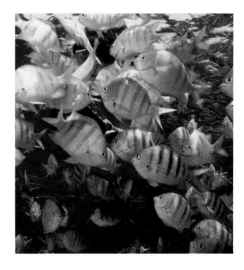

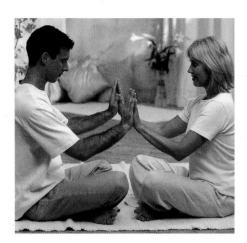

intoxicants, 71
Irlen, Helen, 62–3

Jackson, Carol, 18–19

kitchens, 23

landscapes, 10–11
Liberman, Jacob, 75
light, 54, 55, 56–7, 74–5
living rooms, 24–5
Lorber, Jacob, 74

magenta, 60–1
magic, 74
meditation, 62, 90, 92–3
migraine, 63

names, 85
nature, 10–13
nervous system, 54, 55
night, 56

offices, 21, 27
oils, essential, 79
orange, 36–7
    chakras, 87, 88
    colour visualization, 91
    commercial use of colour, 20
    crystals, 80
    foods, 68
    light, 56
    single colour assessment, 60–1

Pancoast, Dr Seth, 74–5
Paracelsus, 78
personality types, 19
pineal gland, 54, 55, 57, 88–9
pink, 49
    colour visualization, 91

crystals, 81
    single colour assessment, 60–1
pituitary gland, 54, 55, 89
plants, 12, 56, 78–9
Plato, 84
Platonic solids, 84, 85

rainbow breathing, 91
rainbow diet, 66–71
reading difficulties, 62–3
red, 32–3
    chakras, 87, 88
    colour visualization, 90, 91
    commercial use of colour, 20
    crystals, 80
    cultural variations, 14–15
    double-colour healing, 82
    flowers, 79
    foods, 67
    light, 56
    meditation, 62, 93
    single colour assessment, 60–1
rods and cones, 54–5
root chakra, 87

sacral chakra, 87
sacred shapes, 84
St John's wort, 78
Scotopic Sensitivity Syndrome (SSS), 62–3
Seasonal Affective Disorder (SAD), 57
shape and colour, 84–5
single colour assessment, 60–1
solar plexus chakra, 87
Spitter, Dr Harry R., 75
spring colours, 18
Steiner, Rudolph, 74
studies, 27
summer colours, 18–19
Sun, Howard and Dorothy, 85
sunlight, 54, 55, 56–7, 74
symbolism, cultural variations, 14–15
synaesthesia, 85
syntonics, 75

tartans, 16
tattva system, 84, 92–3
Third Eye, 88–9
throat chakra, 88
Tibetan Buddhism, 90, 92
transparent crystals, 80, 81
Turner, J.M.W., 74
turquoise, 48
    double-colour healing, 83
    single colour assessment, 60–1

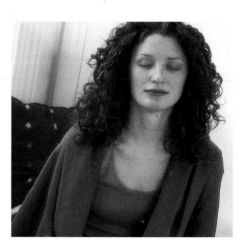

ultra-violet light, 56

Vedic texts, 86, 88
vegetables, 66–71
vibrational healing, 76–7
violet, 44–5
    chakras, 88, 89
    crystals, 81
    double-colour healing, 83
    foods, 71
    single colour assessment, 60–1
visualization, 62, 90–1
Vitale, Barbara Meister, 63

white, 46–7
    chakras, 87, 88, 89
    commercial use of colour, 20
    crystals, 81
    cultural variations, 14–15
    light, 56
    meditation, 93
    single colour assessment, 60–1
winter, 14, 57
winter colours, 19
work, 21
workrooms, 27

yellow, 34–5
    chakras, 87, 88
    colour visualization, 90
    commercial use of colour, 20
    crystals, 80
    double-colour healing, 82
    and exams, 62
    flowers, 78
    foods, 69
    light, 56
    meditation, 92
    single colour assessment, 60–1
yoga, 86–9